Health, Risk and News

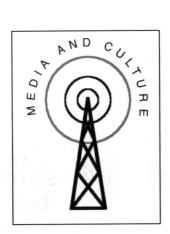

Sut Jhally & Justin Lewis
General Editors

Vol. 9

PETER LANG
New York • Washington, D.C./Baltimore • Bern
Frankfurt am Main • Berlin • Brussels • Vienna • Oxford

Health, Risk and News

PETER LANG
New York • Washington, D.C./Baltimore • Bern
Frankfurt am Main • Berlin • Brussels • Vienna • Oxford

Library of Congress Cataloging-in-Publication Data

Boyce, Tammy.
Health, risk and news: the MMR vaccine and the media / Tammy Boyce.
p. cm. — (Media and culture; v. 9)
Includes bibliographical references and index.
1. Health in mass media. 2. Mass media—Great Britain. 3. MMR vaccine—Great
Britain. 4. Autism—Great Britain. 5. Health risk assessment—
Great Britain. I. Title. II. Series: Media & culture (New York, N.Y.); v. 9.
P96.H432G73   614.4'241—dc22   2007028799
ISBN 978-0-8204-8838-7
ISSN 1098-4208

Bibliographic information published by **Die Deutsche Bibliothek**.
Die Deutsche Bibliothek lists this publication in the "Deutsche
Nationalbibliografie"; detailed bibliographic data is available
on the Internet at http://dnb.ddb.de/.

Cover design by Sophie Appel

The paper in this book meets the guidelines for permanence and durability
of the Committee on Production Guidelines for Book Longevity
of the Council of Library Resources.

Printed in the United States of America

Contents

Acknowledgments

Many, many, many warm words of thanks to the colleagues, friends and family who have, in various quantities and guises, encouraged me, challenged my ideas and generally helped me along the way. Particular thanks to Justin Lewis and Jenny Kitzinger, who both gave a great deal of their time and advice. Special thanks also to Karin Wahl-Jorgensen, Emma Hughes, Sanna Inthorn, Harry Collins, Rob Evans, JOMEC technicians and Sophie Appel at Peter Lang.

Many of those involved in the MMR/autism story have been patient and understanding and were ready to answer my queries: Fiona Fox, Dr. Helen Bedford, Dr. David Elliman, Vivienne Parry and Dr. Mike Fitzpatrick. Many thanks to the mothers who shared their views in the focus groups. For motivation and showing me hard work pays off, thanks to Kati, Sandrine, Anna, Amélie and all. My family and friends have been patient in understanding the pressures on my time and deserve a special mention for this patience: Julie, Kadin, Owen, Ieuan, Sally, Gloria, Rob, Kim, Melodie, Ankë, Mari, Roger, Andrew, Yan, Seema and Katie.

Linda, all of those years we spent shouting at the tv and being outraged at newspapers, who knew it would be so useful! You were my first media studies teacher; many thanks. Siân, much gratitude for support, patience and motivation and all conversations about vaccines. A torment and delight!

Abbreviations

BMA	British Medical Association
CMO	Chief Medical Officer (Dr. Liam Donaldson)
DoH	Department of Health
GMC	General Medical Council
GP	General Practitioner (Family doctor)
HPA	Health Protection Agency
JABS	Justice, Awareness and Basic Support
JCVI	Joint Council for Vaccinations and Immunisation
MMR	Measles, mumps and rubella vaccine
MRC	Medical Research Council
NAS	National Autistic Society
NHS	National Health Service
PHLS	Public Health Laboratory Service (now Health Protection Agency)
RCGP	Royal College of General Practitioners
RCN	Royal College of Nursing
RCPCH	Royal College of Paediatrics and Child Health
RI	Royal Institution
SMC	Science Media Centre
WHO	World Health Organisation

CHAPTER ONE

Introduction

For parents in the United Kingdom, whether or not to have the measles, mumps and rubella vaccine is one of the most significant decisions they believe they will make about their child's health. No longer simply another step in the childhood vaccination schedule, since 1998 the MMR vaccine and the alleged link to autism has become an intense topic of debate for parents, grandparents and all those caring for children. The British media have not simply stood by and reported this story; instead they have been active participants in keeping the MMR vaccine at the top of the news agenda. This book seeks to understand why the MMR/autism debate received such significant coverage in the British media whilst remaining uncontroversial in the rest of the world. What is it about this story that makes it so appealing to the British media?

The story of the MMR vaccine and its links to autism has one protagonist: Dr. Andrew Wakefield. He made his first allegations that the MMR vaccine might be linked to autism in 1995 and in subsequent years the UK media have consistently covered the story. Whilst working on a project about science, the public and the media (Hargreaves et al. 2003) I watched, read and listened to hundreds of stories about the MMR/autism story. With no research actually linking the MMR vaccine to autism, I struggled to understand why this story was so often on the front pages or on the television news. Media coverage did not comprise of one monolithic message 'MMR is unsafe' however, the more MMR/autism stories I consumed, the more it appeared that the pro-MMR side was unsuccessful at defending or promoting the MMR vaccine. The media coverage suggested there were numerous Greek choruses criticising and questioning the safety of the MMR vaccine versus a few weak, mumbling stragglers defending it. I was left with a number of questions in my quest to understand why the MMR vaccine/autism link received so much media attention:

- Why did the story attract such consistent media attention when few events (new research, political statements) happened? What was making this story so attractive to journalists?
- Why was it always the *same* small pool of sources making the *same* arguments supporting Dr. Andrew Wakefield yet scores of different sources were making a variety of arguments questioning his findings? Were there really so few anti-MMR sources? And why did journalists not see the discrepancy between the number of scientists stating the safety of the vaccine versus those accusing it of being dangerous?
- Why was this medical/science story so often covered by non-science/health specialists? Why did so many different journalists cover the story?

But the foremost question raised was *who was responsible for promoting and defending the MMR vaccine and why weren't they doing it?*

The antagonistic coverage of the MMR vaccine seemed inconsistent in light of positive public attitudes towards vaccinations in the UK. Childhood vaccinations are not compulsory, yet vaccination rates usually approach the recommended level for herd immunity of 95%.[1] The UK government uses various methods to encourage uptake; the two main methods are either through their GP or via public service advertisements. GPs also receive a financial incentive because 'spontaneous parental compliance was not considered sufficient, in itself, to ensure targets being met' (Rogers and Pilgrim 1995: 73).[2] In other countries, such as the USA, childhood vaccinations are compulsory and children are not able to attend publicly funded schools unless they have been vaccinated or have valid medical reasons not to be.

A Short History of the Measles, Mumps and Rubella Vaccine — The 'MMR Vaccine'

The measles, mumps and rubella triple vaccine (MMR), first approved in the USA in 1971, is widely used in over 90 countries. The MMR vaccine was introduced into the United Kingdom in 1988 by the Conservative government and parents did not hesitate to have their children vaccinated with the triple vaccine. In one year, one million children were inoculated. From the introduction of the triple vaccine in 1988 until 1997, MMR immunisation levels remained over 90%. In

1996 the UK government introduced a second MMR vaccination to 'boost' protection against measles after research found it increased the level of immunity in the vaccinated population (Peltola et al. 1994). The MMR triple jab is usually given between the ages of 12 and 15 months and the booster between 4 and 6 years. Both vaccines are provided free of charge by the National Health Service (NHS). Single vaccines are currently available from private health care clinics at the cost of hundreds of pounds.[3] Single vaccines are only available on the NHS if a child has already received one of the vaccines in a single form.[4]

The uptake of the MMR vaccine started to decline in late 1997, then stabilised during 1999 and 2000 and declined again in 2001. The national MMR vaccine uptake continued to fall in the following three years. Uptake is uneven across the UK, with some areas reaching the level required for herd immunity whilst in other areas, like London, levels dropped below 70%. The uptake started to slowly rise in 2005 and at the time of writing, the national vaccination rate continues to increase but uptake remains below 80%, with wide variation across the UK.[5]

The alleged link between the MMR vaccine and autism began in the mid-1990s. Dr. Andrew Wakefield, then an adult gastroenterologist at London's Royal Free Hospital, published a short study in the British medical journal *The Lancet* claiming a link between measles and Crohn's disease (Ekbom et al. 1994). In 1995 Wakefield first suggested there might be a link between *measles* and autism in a short piece in *The Lancet* (Thompson et al. 1995). Not proving a link, the paper's vague conclusion stated the 'measles virus may play a part in the development not only of Crohn's disease but also of ulcerative colitis'; the vaccine did not figure in the conclusions. These early allegations received little media attention and were only picked up by the *Guardian, Daily Mail* and *The Times* and covered for just one day.

Wakefield's February 1998 research catapulted his theory to the top of the news agenda. This research, written by Wakefield and colleagues at the Royal Free Hospital (Wakefield et al. 1998) and again published in *The Lancet,* was based on a case study of 12 children with an unusual bowel syndrome. The discussion paper argued that eight of the 12 children under study had a 'pattern of intestinal abnormalities and regressive development disorder' and this might represent a new syndrome which they labelled 'autistic entercolitis'. The research alleged to have discovered traces of the *measles virus* in the children's guts. They regarded the presence of the virus as *perhaps potentially* relevant in causing autism and inflammatory bowel disease. The published research presented no evidence linking the MMR vaccine to inflammatory bowel disease or to autism; in fact, *the vaccine was not once mentioned in the research.*

Instead, Dr. Wakefield made the allegation against the vaccine at a press conference publicising the *Lancet* research at the Royal Free Hospital. It was also at this press conference that Wakefield raised the point that would leave an imprint on the UK public and provide a rallying cry for parents. He argued that giving children the vaccines in *three separate doses* would be safer – a suggestion not supported by any data produced by Wakefield in this research, nor in subsequent research. In the press conference, the majority of his co-authors openly stated they did not support this suggestion, nor have they in subsequent publications.

The hospital was well aware that Wakefield was going to make these claims in the press conference as these ideas, that the MMR vaccine could potentially be linked to autism and that single vaccines might be a better solution, were discussed in a video news release (VNR) supplied by the publicity department at the Royal Free Hospital. In an extract from the press conference Wakefield openly makes his claims:

> **Interviewer (off screen):** There has been concern recently over any long term effects as a result of the MMR vaccine, are you saying now then that there does appear to be a proven link between the vaccine and the side effects?
>
> **Dr Andrew Wakefield:** No. The work certainly raises a question mark over MMR vaccine, there is no proven link as such and we are seeking to establish whether there is a genuine causal association between the MMR and this syndrome or not. It is our suspicion that there may well be, but that is far from being a causal association that is proven beyond doubt.
>
> **Interviewer:** But if you say there's at least a question mark over it now, should the vaccine continue to be administered while you're investigating?
>
> **Dr Andrew Wakefield:** I think if you asked members of the team that have investigated this they would give you different answers. And I have to say that there is sufficient anxiety in my own mind of the safety, the long term safety of the polyvalent, that is the MMR vaccination in combination, that I think that it should be suspended in favour of the single vaccines, that is continued use of the individual measles, mumps and rubella components.[6]

He repeats this claim about single vaccines a few minutes later:

> **Interviewer:** So you're saying that a parent should still ensure that their child is inoculated but perhaps not with the MMR combined vaccine?
> **Dr Andrew Wakefield:** Again, this was very contentious and you would not get consensus from all members of the group on this, but that is my feeling, that the, the risk of this particular syndrome developing is related to the combined vaccine, the MMR, rather than the single vaccines.

And a third time:

> **Dr Andrew Wakefield:** My opinion, again, is that the monovalent, the single vaccines, measles, mumps and rubella, are likely in this context to be safer than the polyvalent vaccine.

During the press conference the Dean of the Royal Free's medical school, Dr. Arie Zuckerman, attempted to limit the damage of Wakefield's accusation by stating he did not believe Wakefield's evidence justified ceasing to use the MMR vaccine. But as indicated above, the interview with Wakefield (the lead author of the study and an employee of the Royal Free) in the hospital's *own* VNR stated that the MMR vaccine was potentially dangerous: not once, but three times. Zuckerman's words were too late, and indeed, the Royal Free Hospital's position was confusing and contradictory to those journalists attending the press conference.

Media coverage of this infamous 1998 press conference has developed its own folklore. The stories that arose out of this press conference were not the panic-inducing or contentious stories that were seen in subsequent years. At the time, Wakefield's co-authors even stated that 'the media response has in fact been notably balanced, with almost all reports endorsing current immunisation schedules, until further evidence is forthcoming' (Murch et al. 1998: 9106). On 27 February 1998 the press conference appeared on the front pages of *The Guardian* and *The Independent*, but was not even covered in *The Sun* and only on pages 13 and 14 in the *Daily Mail*. After this initial flurry of articles, coverage was muted and remained so until 2001 (see Table 1.1). Coverage reached a peak in 2002 and still continues to receive significant coverage in the UK press.

Wakefield's next publication was in the *American Journal of Gastroenterology* (Wakefield et al. 2000), a journal with a much smaller circulation and therefore less prestigious than *The Lancet*. Wakefield's research eventually attempted to link the measles *virus* with bowel disease. Failing to provide evidence, Wakefield *suggested* (but did not 'prove' with research[8]) that the MMR vaccine might be the problem

Table 1.1 Number of articles containing 'MMR' in UK/US national newspapers[7]

Year	# stories UK Papers	England and Wales MMR rate	# stories USA papers	USA MMR rate	Selected events and publications
1995	10	92%	11	90%	- Thompson et al. 1995 - First Wakefield article in national UK paper (*Sunday Times*)
1996	18	92%	3	91%	~
1997	34	91%	7	90%	- Labour govt. elected
1998	122	88%	7	92%	- Wakefield et al. in *The Lancet*
1999	133	88%	9	92%	~
2000	136	87%	18	91%	- Wakefield et al. 2000
2001	764	84%	26	92%	~
2002	1257	82%	31	92%	- *Panorama* aired - Leo Blair at MMR vaccination age (May) - Wakefield leaves Royal Free Hospital
2003	707	80%	16	93%	~
2004	700	81%	25	93%	- Brian Deer Channel 4 documentary and *Sunday Times* articles; - mumps outbreaks in university students UK front page news
2005	358	84%	22	92%	~
2006	386	NA	16	NA	- First death from measles in UK since MMR introduced; - Scientists write a joint letter to UK media to 'draw a line under the question of any association between the MMR vaccine and autism' - GMC investigation into Wakefield begins - Chancellor Gordon Brown's child has MMR

for this. The reason? Giving the three vaccines in one does would 'overwhelm' the immune system and potentially act as a 'trigger' for autism and inflammatory bowel disease.

In 2002 two events brought the MMR vaccine onto the British national news agenda. The BBC programme *Panorama* ('How safe is MMR?' broadcast 3 February 2002, BBC 1) examined Wakefield's latest research published in *Molecular Pathology*, a medical journal with a small circulation (Uhlmann et al. 2002).[9] The paper claimed to confirm an association between the presence of the measles virus and gut pathology in children with a developmental disorder. Again, there was no mention of the MMR vaccine. The paper claimed to show a link between gut pathology and the measles virus but did not differentiate whether the virus was naturally occurring or a result of the triple or single vaccine. As will be shown, the media coverage failed to address this key difference – that this research did not *prove* or even examine a link between the *MMR vaccine* and autism, but was making another hypothesis altogether.

Numerous measles cases in London[10] and North England was the second reason for the high level of media attention in February 2002. The appearance of measles in middle-class areas provided journalists with a different angle to report the MMR/autism story. After 2002, media coverage of the MMR vaccine declined. In 2003 and 2004, coverage was still fairly substantial as the UK media continued to cover Wakefield's new research and claims. By 2005 there was a further drop in media coverage. The number of articles increases slightly in 2006 firstly because of the General Medical Council's (the doctor's disciplinary body) decision to bring charges of misconduct against Wakefield and, secondly, because of Wakefield's decision to sue journalist Brian Deer (the case was thrown out of court in January 2007 and Wakefield subsequently paid damages to Deer).

Wakefield resigned from his post at the Royal Free Hospital in 2002, although some, including the editor of *The Lancet*, argue this was done 'under considerable pressure' (Horton 2004a: 28). Since his departure Wakefield has worked for a variety of organisations including the private health care company Direct Health 2000[11] and he wa 'associated' with the International Child Development Resource Center in Florida, although his specific role was unclear.[12] He is currently executive director of Thoughtful House in Texas, a school and clinic treating children with autism. Supporters of Wakefield created the charity Visceral to fund his work and Visceral plays an important role in publicising the MMR/autism link. The public relations agency Bell Pottinger represents both Visceral and Dr. Wakefield. Bell Pottinger is a large and established PR agency in the UK and has represented figures like Margaret Thatcher. Under their tutelage, Wakefield only speaks to a selected group of UK journalists, most of whom support his claim of a link between the MMR vaccine and autism.

Almost all of Wakefield's co-authors from the 1998 *Lancet* research have distanced themselves from the MMR/autism hypothesis. In October 2003 Dr. Simon Murch, one of the authors of the 1998 *Lancet* paper, blatantly positioned himself as far away from Wakefield as he possibly could in a letter to *The Lancet*:

> That any reports that characterise gut inflammation in autistic children are reported in the media as supporting the ideas that MMR is causative is deeply frustrating, since it is simply not so...There is now unequivocal evidence that MMR is not a risk factor for autism – this statement is not spin or medical conspiracy, but reflects an unprecedented volume of medical study on a worldwide basis.
>
> (Murch 2003: 1498)

In an interview on the BBC *Today* programme on the day this letter was published, Murch explained he wrote the letter because of his worry of a measles epidemic occurring as a result of the falling vaccination rates. Wakefield was interviewed immediately afterwards and accused Murch of writing the letter for professional reputation reasons and Wakefield then dropped the accusation that the Joint Council for Vaccinations and Immunisation (JCVI) was withholding evidence that supported the MMR/autism link (Wakefield 2003). The following day a member of the JCVI told me she was 'amazed' by Wakefield's accusation and that the JCVI were unaware of any research. Since then, no evidence has been revealed that supports Wakefield's claim of the JCVI witholding evidence nor has he made the accusation again.

Subsequent to the publication of Wakefield's *Lancet* article in 1998, UK policy-makers, politicians, clinicians and the Department of Health have all been forced to defend a vaccination policy that is, for the most part, uncontroversial in the rest of the Western world. Various accusations have been made against the MMR vaccine in the USA, Sweden and Germany but they failed to have a serious impact on national vaccination rates. In 1993 Denmark's MMR uptake fell after a television programme questioned its safety but rates rose again after this acute media attention (Begg et al. 1998: 561).[13] During the period the MMR uptake fell in the UK, levels of other vaccinations remain unaffected, signalling that parents are not rejecting the idea of vaccinations in general, but only the MMR vaccine.

One month after the publication of Wakefield's 1998 paper the Chief Medical Officer asked the Medical Research Council (MRC) to convene an ad hoc group to consider the available data relating to a possible link between the MMR vaccine, autism and inflammatory bowel conditions. Over 30 experts met to discuss Wakefield's findings. They reported in December 2001 and concluded there was no evidence of a causal link (MRC 2001).

The medical community's response to Wakefield has been two-fold. Firstly, they countered Wakefield's claims with numerous pieces of research. Secondly, they sought to understand why vaccination rates fell and concentrated on the media's role in this decline and, for the most part, failed to analyse their own actions (or lack thereof). The majority of research examining Wakefield's theories is epidemiological and refutes the MMR/autism link.[14] One of the criticisms of these large epidemiological studies is that they would not reveal a problem with the vaccine if the risk only affected a tiny subset of the population. (In epidemiological studies the risk needs to be common enough to be visible in large population studies.) This is one of Wakefield's main criticisms of the research that attempts to refute his allegations – he argues epidemiological studies are not able to 'disprove' his research. Nonetheless, the weight of existing scientific evidence unequivocally suggests that the MMR vaccine is not linked to autism. Donald and Muthu's (2002) review of research suggests that all the credible evidence refutes any link and that there is still, to date, no empirical data linking the vaccine to autism (see also the Cochrane review of evidence, Demicheli et al. 2005). The cause of autism remains unknown, but most research links it to environmental or genetic factors.[15]

As well as responding to Wakefield's scientific claims, scientists have also analysed why parents have been so quick to accept his theories, with most research holding the media responsible. For example, Evans et al.'s research with parents argued 'media reports about MMR had affected most parents' immunisation decisions, except for those few who were already committed to their views, being either strongly pro or strongly anti-immunisation' (2001: 909). Similarly, in a longitudinal study of vaccination rates, Ramsay et al. showed that awareness of and perceived safety in the MMR vaccine fell after significant periods of media interest but rose again once media interest fell away (2002: 914-915).[16] Mason and Donnelly (2000) examined coverage of the MMR/autism story in the local Swansea paper *The South Wales Evening Post (SWEP)* and compared the Swansea MMR uptake rates with the vaccination rates across Wales. Since 1997, coverage of the MMR vaccine in the *SWEP* has primarily challenged the safety of the triple jab and supported Wakefield's theories. Many stories, predominantly written by one journalist, covered the experiences of parents who claimed their child's autism was linked to the MMR vaccine. Mason and Donnelly found the MMR uptake in the Swansea area declined by 13.6% compared to 2.4% in the rest of Wales, 'a statistically significant greater decline in the distribution area of the *SWEP*' (2000: 473). They admit their conclusion cannot claim a *causal relationship* but they do suggest the newspaper 'has had a measurable and unhelpful impact over and above any adverse national publicity' (ibid.).

In addition to Wakefield's scientific research, another event contributed to how this story has evolved. In the mid-1990s, before the 1998 *Lancet* paper, a group of parents initiated a legal case against the vaccine manufacturers claiming the MMR vaccine had caused their children's autism.[17] The parents received Legal Aid Board (LAB) funding from the government. Wakefield was not an impartial observer of this legal case. As would later be revealed, he was a member of the scientific team that helped to secure the LAB funding. This participation in the legal case against the MMR vaccine raised a serious potential conflict of interest as he failed to acknowledge his participation in this legal case in his publications. When this issue came to light, Wakefield was criticised by his scientific colleagues and his participation in the legal case would also mark the beginning of his downfall. It led to the General Medical Council investigation of his work and the possibility of Wakefield being unable to practice medicine in the UK (at the time of publication this case has yet to be decided).

These revelations came about because of the work of independent investigative journalist Brian Deer. In early 2004 Deer (2004a, 2004b) published evidence in the British newspaper *The Sunday Times* claiming Wakefield had not disclosed funding he received from the Legal Aid Board at the time of submitting his 1998 *Lancet* publication. Wakefield had therefore failed to declare a 'conflict of interest'. Because of this revelation, *The Lancet* partially retracted the 1998 publication in an editorial statement (Horton 2004b). Deer's second allegation appeared in the November 2004 Channel 4 series *Dispatches* (broadcast 18 November). Among a number of revelations, Deer revealed that a few months before the 1998 *Lancet* article, Wakefield had secured patents for a new single measles vaccine thus Wakefield would potentially financially benefit if the UK returned to single vaccines. Both of Deer's allegations seriously raised the possibility of a financial conflict of interest.[18]

At the time when Wakefield was making his accusations about the MMR vaccine and autism, a group of parents created JABS, Justice, Awareness and Basic Support. JABS is a campaigning and support group for parents claiming their children had been damaged by the MMR vaccine.[19] JABS has two main objectives: to secure recognition and financial compensation for their damaged children and 'to make the vaccine system safer so other children are not damaged'.[20] Jackie Fletcher, the founder of JABS, believes her son's autism was a result of the MMR vaccine. Fletcher set up the group after meeting other families in her local hospital 'who were also saying that their child had had fits shortly after the MMR'. The group initially used the local media to find other parents, and in their local area alone (a small town in England), they found 30 other families making similar claims against the MMR vaccine. By 2004 Fletcher stated JABS had over 2,000 families on their register. Fletcher herself had no scientific or media background, but over the past ten years, she has become literate in biology, vaccines, epidemiology and public relations.

JABS was part of a delegation that met with the Labour government five months after it was elected in 1997. Tessa Jowell, then Public Health Minister, met a deputation that marked a significant step forward for the anti-MMR campaign. The group included key anti-MMR figures such as solicitor Richard Barr, Dr. Andrew Wakefield and Jackie Fletcher. The date of the meeting is important as the group met *before* Wakefield's *Lancet* 1998 publication, confirming that the government was aware of Wakefield's claims between the MMR vaccine and autism. It was at this stage that JABS decided to engage more closely with the media. Wakefield and JABS understood from an early stage that media coverage is 'crucial to the constitution of authority in the knowledge structure of society' (Ericson et al. 1989: 23). Groups compete to appear in the media not only to make themselves credible (in the eyes of both the public and policy-makers) but also to raise their profile, highlight a particular issue and increase financial support.

In 2004, instead of the measles outbreaks many had predicted as a result of the falling MMR vaccination uptake, mumps outbreaks were a common occurrence in universities and A-Level colleges. As a result, the MMR vaccine was offered to thousands of university students.[21] This time is was not the autism link providing the angle for these front page headlines, but the return of measles, mumps and rubella; 'Mumps hits universities Vaccination campaign as cases jump' (*Daily Telegraph* 2.11.04), 'Mumps hits students at medical college' (*Evening Standard*, 14.12.04) and 'War on Mumps' (*The Mirror* 3.12.04). In 2005 and 2006 mumps and measles outbreaks continued across the UK in a range of ages.[22]

An Earlier Vaccine Scare: The Pertussis Controversy

Prior to the attention given to the MMR vaccine, another vaccine was the subject of intense media attention in the UK. In the 1970s the pertussis vaccine (whooping cough, taken as part of the DTP vaccine – diphtheria, tetanus and pertussis) was the subject of critical research by Professor John Wilson (Kulenkampff et al. 1974). The research suggested that the vaccine may cause rare cases of neurological injury. The research claimed to attribute 36 neurological reactions to whole-cell pertussis. Like the MMR vaccine, the research only signalled problems with one element of the triple vaccine, the pertussis vaccine.

Similar to Dr. Wakefield, Professor Wilson made many of his claims via the media and not through peer-reviewed publications. In April 1974 he claimed on the prime-time ITV documentary series *This Week* that there was an 'established' link between the vaccine and neurological injury, claiming to have seen 80 affected patients (Deer 1998). Retrospective research shows the medical profession was unprepared for 'the storm of media publicity that soon followed' (Baker 2003: 4004). In the UK, vaccination rates plummeted, falling from 77% to 33%.[23] Epidemics followed, and between 1977 and 1979, 27 people died from whooping cough and there were 17 cases of permanent brain damage (Fitzpatrick 2004: 25). The health minister and Prince William were vaccinated during this period 'amidst great publicity' (Baker 2003: 4005), but otherwise, politicians were silent on the issue. The pertussis vaccine was not withdrawn throughout this period and confidence in this triple vaccine was eventually restored. Health professionals concluded that confidence was restored due to published research demonstrating the vaccine was safe and provided essential protection against the three diseases. In addition, a series of failed compensation claims led the public to believe the case against the DTP vaccine was groundless (Gangarosa 1998, Fitzpatrick 2004).

Scientists and health professionals have carefully examined the lessons to be learned from this earlier vaccine controversy. Several commentators point out that it could have had lessons for the MMR crisis not least because the pertussis scare and the MMR/autism story have many similarities: the heightened media interest, falling vaccination rates and a vocal group of parents. The majority of research by scientists about the pertussis and MMR vaccine scares blames the media for paying too much attention to the claims of a small number of scientists and what have been labelled 'anti-vaccine' parents.[24] Scientists were aware of the role parents played in sustaining the DTP crisis (Baker 2003: 4003) and that the existence of these parental groups led to a decline in vaccine uptakes. Whilst this research shows scientists were aware of the power of these groups, they do not appear to have formulated ideas on how to challenge these parents.

Health Communication

Part of the reason why health care professionals have not learned from previous vaccination scares is their belief that if the public had enough information they would make healthy choices; this is the basis of health education campaigns (see, for instance, Rimal et al. 1999, Logan 1991). Doctors and health care workers wish the public would listen to their facts and arguments and this will then lead to an improvement in their own health. There is a dichotomy between health educators, who see the media as a teaching tool, and journalists, who 'consider themselves primarily reporters rather than educators' (Lantz and Lanier 2002: 1306). Contributing to the complexity of these competing roles is the role of scientists, who increasingly turn to the media to publicise their research and inform the public. All three of these groups—health professionals, scientists and journalists—have different reasons for transmitting information to the public and this can have complex and confusing effects on the audience. The effect of these competing roles are central to what this book explores—what messages were in the media, who was trying to get messages into the media and what audiences were doing with all of this information.

Method and Outline

The following chapters are based on research that analyses the production, content and reception of the MMR/autism story. The content analysis studies UK television, radio and the quality and popular press, from 1 February to 15 September 2002. The sample covers periods when the story was at the top of the news agenda and when it fell further down. The two television news programmes with the largest audiences in the UK are analysed, the weekday BBC 6:00 evening news and ITV 6:30 evening news. The newspaper sample uses the Lexis-Nexis database to study five dailies: *The Guardian, Daily Telegraph, Daily Mail, The Sun, Daily Mirror* and four Sunday newspapers, *Mail on Sunday, Sunday Times, News of the World* and *The Observer*.[25] The BBC Radio 4 morning news programme *Today* was selected because of its large audience (approximately 8-10 million listeners) and its influential role on the wider news agenda. Highlights archived on the internet were analysed.[26]

All those items that contained the term 'MMR' were analysed in detail. The stories were then divided into four categories: primary theme, secondary theme, single-mention and letters. The criterion for inclusion in the primary theme group was discussion of the MMR vaccination in more than two sentences. A total of 513 items were identified of which 285 had MMR as the primary theme. These 285 newspaper, television and radio stories are the subject of the content analysis and are all merged together in the category of 'primary theme stories' (see Table 1.2).

The audience analysis draws on the results of two nationally representative audience surveys of over 1,000 respondents and four focus groups held in South Wales.

The production analysis comprised of 19 interviews with sources and journalists. Journalists selected for interview were those who had presented or written stories about the MMR vaccine in each media organisation studied. Eight national journalists were interviewed of which six were science or health specialists, one columnist and one general news correspondent (see Box 1.1).

Table 1.2 Media sample: Stories analysed
1 February-15 September 2002

Media	No. stories
Daily Mail	56
The Sun	51
The Mirror	43
Guardian	35
Daily Telegraph	30
Sunday Times	12
Mail on Sunday	11
News of the World	10
Observer	8
Today Programme	15
ITV Evening News	8
BBC Evening News	6
Total	285

Box 1.1 Journalists interviewed

Representatives from:

- *The Guardian*   -   *Daily Telegraph*
- *ITV News*   -   *Mail on Sunday*
- *Sunday Times*   -   *The Mirror*
- *Today* Programme   -   Freelance journalists

Sources interviewed were selected for two reasons, either they were common sources found in the media coverage or they were well-known medical or scientific organisations representing doctors, nurses and scientists. A total of 12 sources were interviewed (see Box 1.2). The sample is also informed by a number of conferences, meetings and debates I attended, where I spoke to a number of sources including representatives from the Public Health Laboratory Service (later the Health Protection Agency), GPs, Visceral, Sense (the rubella charity) and a range of journalists.

I requested an interview with Dr. Wakefield and contacted him via his charity Visceral but he declined to be interviewed.[27]

Box 1.2 Sources interviewed

Representatives from:

- Department of Health — Medical Research Council
- Science Media Centre — British Medical Association
- Royal College of General Practitioners
- Royal College of Nursing — Member of Parliament
- Royal College of Paediatrics and Child Health
- Royal Free Hospital — Liberal Democrats
- National Autistic Society — JABS

The following 8 chapters discuss key themes that the MMR/autism story raises for the reporting of health, science and risk stories. Chapter 2 provides an overview of the reporting of health and risk and examines how these themes fit into the MMR/autism story. Chapter 3 continues to examine ideas around risk and health and argues current categories of news values do not adequately address the news values of risk, health and science stories. In Chapter 4 the concept of balance is questioned in the reporting of health, science and risk stories. Chapters 5 and 6 examine the relationship between journalists and their sources. Chapter 5 looks at the sources selected by journalists and compares this with the actions of the sources and the attitudes of journalists. Chapter 6 is a detailed analysis of the actions of the pro-MMR health and science sources, examining their efforts and their lack of success at influencing how this story was told. Both of these chapters open up new ideas about researching sources. Chapter 7 considers the role expertise played in selecting and presenting sources and proposes more attention be paid to "expert-sources" when studying sources. How the MMR/autism story affected audiences is examined in Chapter 8, analysing the sources of information and rationales used by parents when making their MMR vaccination decision. The conclusion brings together these ideas and considers the lessons to be learned from this story – lessons for sources, journalists, the health profession, media studies scholars and audiences.

Reporting Health, Science and Risk

I n the post-World War Two era the health of the average citizen in the deliberately developed world continues to improve and life expectancies increase. At the same time, health stories have become more prominent and profuse in the Western media. Healthier citizens who live longer are reading more often about a wider range of health risks and scares.

The public have not always been so consumed with their health. In 1968 only one in ten claimed to be concerned about their health. Thirty years later this figure rose to one in two (Le Fanu 1999: 28). Surveys show that both British and American adults are more likely to read newspaper stories with headlines concerning medical issues compared to other subjects (Durant in Lupton 1998: 194). The Western media continue to pay greater attention to health, in an era when our health is at its best.

As the West's concern for health was expanding, the media and information universe was also growing; there are more television and radio channels, longer newspapers, more magazines and of course, the ever-expanding internet. As the media grows, so has the number of journalists and specialist correspondents. Tunstall (1971) discusses the growth of science correspondents occurring after the atomic bomb in 1945 and the number of health correspondents have also increased since the 1980s as Western audiences become more interested in taking care of their own health. The growth of specialist health and science correspondents is also related to the massive growth in personal health care products and private health care (Tunstall explored this issue as early as 1971 when he could not have foreseen the explosion in private health care in the UK).

However, the changing nature of health coverage is not simply down to increased coverage. There is some disagreement as to why this change has occurred. Some researchers argue journalists are not simply reproducing the findings in medical or science journals but are 'now more involved in exposing the hypocrisy of science, medicine and professionalism' (Reed 2001: 290). Others disagree that journalists are always this sceptical, arguing that in spite of the increasing coverage of health and medical issues, 'medical definitions and perceptions still prevail and squeeze out more contentious, oppositional viewpoints which...look at the politics of health' (Karpf 1988: 2). Lupton agrees, stating medical definitions in the media dominate, arguing that health news stories still tend to use doctors as figures of authority (1998: 203). Coverage of health stories is not one-dimensional; it is also influenced by the topic and media outlet. The image of doctors and scientists is fragmented and now encompasses both supportive and critical depictions.

Simultaneous to the media expansion and the increasing attention to health is the idea that we live in a world of ever-expanding risks and awareness of these risks. With a public more attentive to potential health disasters lurking in their everyday lives, journalists have more opportunities to appeal to these interests and fears. Everyday objects have become dangerous: meat in the Bovine Spongiform Encephalopathy (BSE) crisis, eggs and salmonella, the birth-control pill, tea, coffee and an assortment of foods accused of causing cancer and then not causing cancer (see, for example, Seale 2002, Langer 1998, Le Fanu 1999: 28). Coverage of risks has increased, coverage of health has increased and coverage of science has increased – none of this without criticisms from scientists and health professionals. This chapter considers four aspects of health and science coverage: the most common criticisms of health and science reporting, the role of specialist correspondents, the impact of peer review and, finally, the enduring influence of the BSE crisis on contemporary reporting of health and science stories in the UK.

Typical Accusations of Health and Science Coverage

Scientists and health professionals' common complaints stem from their belief that the media do not reflect the views of mainstream science. Their criticisms of the media are consistent: the media are sensationalist, irresponsible or simply ill-informed (Seale 2002 and Allan 2002 provide good overviews). This is not a new phenomenon. As early as 1977 the UK Royal Commission on the Press criticised science and medical coverage for 'mistakes, premature publicity, miscon-struction, superficiality, selectivity (e.g., 'good news is no news'), sen-sationalism, betrayal of professional confidentiality (and an) excess of anti-science stories' (Seymour-Ure 1977: 51). Ten years later, Dorothy Nelkin's observations on science in the news in the USA concurred, finding coverage of science tended to 'oversimplify, extrematise and therefore distort the true nature of scientific research and content of scientific findings' (in Seale 2002: 52). The following section outlines the main criticisms made by health professionals and scientists: the excessive focus on controversies, in/accuracy, excessive certainty and the dependency on binary oppositions. Each of these issues is then mapped on to the MMR/autism story.

Focus on Controversies

One of the most common complaints made by scientists is that jour-nalists concentrate too much on controversy when reporting science, health and risk stories. Scientists' accusation is that the media do not simply report controversies; they play 'an active role in shaping and even constructing controversy' (Mazur 1981: 114). Some researchers are sceptical of the science community's claims that media coverage of science emphasises controversies, arguing this view of the media 'stems simply from a view of what coverage should have contained and what emphasis it should have adopted' (Dornan 1999: 187). Sci-ence itself is inherently controversial, being built on experiments, non-linear thinking and hunches. For the media to ignore this side of science would be an unfair representation of the field.

Scientists' main concern is that the media's emphasis on contro-versy will unduly influence attitudes towards science. They worry that the emphasis on controversies in science and health stories, com-bined with the public's lack of background knowledge or understand-ing of the purpose of scientific research, fails to enable the creation of knowledge and instead leads to confusion or apathy. Dearing warns that when 'journalists...seek to portray the most extreme conflicting authoritative positions...the vast majority of mass media audience members lack the ability to evaluate competing claims based on scien-tific criteria' (1994: 343).

When considering the types of messages in the coverage of the MMR/autism story it is clear that there was consistent reporting revolving around the same set of messages and ideas emphasising controversial elements of the story. The most common focus was to emphasise the possible controversial link between the MMR vaccination and autism, included in three-quarters of all stories (see Figure 2.1).

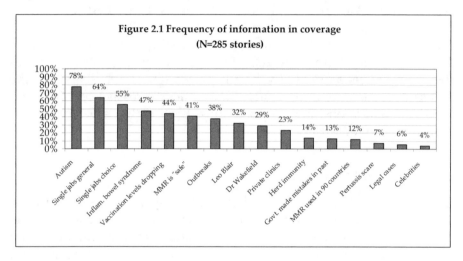

Figure 2.1 Frequency of information in coverage (N=285 stories)

Four of the top five messages all emphasise controversial aspects of the MMR vaccine: the link to autism, single vaccines, that single vaccines should be available on the NHS and the falling vaccination levels.

The fact that the empirical evidence provided by Dr. Wakefield did not involve the vaccine at all (implicating the measles virus, not the MMR vaccine) received very little discussion. The subsequent publicity given to the single vaccines occurred despite there being no empirical evidence to support it. These points matter, because, as the audience chapter will argue, the coverage clearly shaped the way many people understood the issue and led to a loss of confidence in the vaccine in Britain—whilst confidence remains high elsewhere.

Not surprisingly the newspapers which took more of an anti-MMR line were more likely to frame this story as a controversy. *The Sun* and the *Daily Mail* actively campaigned against the MMR vaccine whilst other news outlets adopted a more neutral or even pro-MMR stance. The *Daily Mail* and *The Sun*'s anti-MMR coverage was primarily done by promoting the availability of 'choice' between single vaccines and the MMR vaccine. *The Sun* regularly called for single vaccines to be made available, arguing this in editorials on 5, 6, 7, 9, 11 February, 7, 20 May and 17 June 2002. *Daily Mail* editorials and their columnists also repeatedly called for a choice between single vaccines and the triple MMR vaccine. They did not campaign *against* the MMR vaccine per sé, but repeatedly emphasised the necessity for choice. In doing so, the *Mail* used both subtle and obvious methods to advance their wider agenda of criticising the Labour government. One obvious way of perpetuating the controversy was by labelling the MMR vaccine as 'controversial'; a less subtle way was to mix genres, mainly by merging editorial comment with news. In a front-page article, the *Daily Mail* reports new research by Wakefield and then follows it with this 'Comment' piece. It is unclear whether this is written by the journalist, the *Daily Mail*'s health editor Beezy Marsh, or is an editorial.

> ...COMMENT
>
> WE are witnessing a collapse in public confidence over the Government's soothing reassurances on MMR. Most parents may not be scientists, but they know that some doctors have expressed doubts. And their common sense leads them to wonder whether three powerful injections at the same time might just possibly cause a seriously adverse reaction in a minority of cases. They see the way Tony and Cherie Blair, in a contemptible display of hypocrisy, refuse to give a straight answer on whether or not baby Leo has been given the jab. And they wonder. They wonder why single injections aren't routinely available on the NHS, as they are in France. They wonder why the establishment insists on MMR and refuses to offer a choice. And they wonder why a health service that is supposed to serve the public is treating public concern with something close to contempt. MMR may indeed be perfectly safe. But the behaviour of this Government does not inspire trust.
>
> (6 February 2002)

The *News of the World* (NOTW) also editorialises at the end of a news article about the estimated rise of measles in the UK in 2002.

> ...Panic
>
> What is happening instead is that thousands of parents are going private to protect their children — often being offered expensive single vaccines from abroad that are unsafe. Dr Hilary Jones says: "Some of the clinics cashing in on the panic have been getting their vaccines from Eastern Europe which have been shown to be ineffective."
>
> While Hilary believes MMR is safe, other doctors fear it is dangerous. Peter Mansfield was one of the first GPs to offer single vaccines — and it led to him being hauled before the General Medical Council. He says: "If parents wish

to have single vaccinations there is no reason why they shouldn't. The end result is everybody gets vaccinated." Until the government can produce scientific evidence that MMR never causes autism, surely getting every child vaccinated—however it is done—must be its sole aim. For the sake of hundreds of thousands of children like the tot in our picture—and the 60 who could die this year.

(3 February 2002)

The MMR/autism story was frequently framed and literally labelled as 'controversial' or a 'controversy'. This frequently appeared at the beginning of a story, thus setting a strong frame, such as the following ITV story when the anchor introduces the story:

The controversy surrounding the MMR vaccine deepened today with another suspected outbreak of measles being reported in the North East of England.

(ITV news 4 February 2002)

Overall 40% of all stories included the word 'controversy/controversial' at least once. Each *Mail on Sunday* story includes the word, and in half of the *Daily Mail* stories, the MMR vaccine is labelled as controversial. Journalists refer to both the situation as a 'controversy' and label the MMR vaccine itself as 'controversial'. The use of the word 'controversy' was not the only indication that the story was 'controversial'. Media outlets used various methods to frame the MMR vaccine as controversial. Other ways to emphasise the controversy included repeatedly referring to the decline in public confidence in the vaccine, suggesting not simply that many parents were not vaccinating but explicitly exaggerating the decline. The idea that vaccination levels were falling because of parental anxieties was a point made in 44% of stories even though the majority of parents continued to have their children vaccinated with the MMR vaccine. The *Mail on Sunday* discussed vaccination levels dropping in 82% of their articles. Declining MMR uptake appears less frequently in more neutral or pro-MMR outlets: MMR vaccine rates dropping was in half of *Observer*, BBC television and ITV news stories and down to a quarter of *Mirror* stories.

A number of media reports implied a more dramatic fall in the uptake of the MMR jab. For example, the *Today* programme reported that the MMR vaccine was down to '70% uptake in some areas' (2 February 2002) and the *Daily Mail* reported that 'Uptake of the triple vaccine has fallen to "dangerously low levels" in some areas, according to the Public Health Laboratory Service' (2 February 2002). London historically has a low uptake because of its transient population and the number of new immigrants. However, journalists still used the low uptake in London as a hook. For example, *ITV* News reported that 'in parts of London that figure is down to 65%—meaning only two children in three are having the MMR jab. With so many children left unprotected medical experts fear there is a distinct possibility of a measles epidemic' (5 February 2002). Other media simply made claims without any supporting evidence. *The Sun*, for example, reported:

> ...growing concern of possible links between MMR and autism and bowel disorders have seen a *massive* drop in the number of parents opting for the treatment. Dr Andrew Wakefield made the connection in 1998. No scientists confirmed his findings but many parents say their children changed dramatically after the injection.
>
> (emphasis added, *The Sun* 5 February 2002)

Between 1997 and 2002 the rate of MMR vaccinations had dropped by approximately 6% (it is unclear how much this was due to a lack of confidence in the vaccine). Pro-MMR sources like the Public Health Laboratory Service (PHLS) (subsequently the Health Protection Agency) initially used the declining uptake to try to convince parents to have the MMR vaccine, but after DoH research showed that any publicity about the vaccine led to a decline, they stopped publicising the uptake figures.[1] The uncontroversial point, that most parents were still vaccinating their children with MMR, was rarely covered.[2]

The MMR/autism story was also framed as controversial when journalists intimated Wakefield was a victim, a doctor fighting against the government and establishment science for the truth to be told. *Daily Mail* columnist Quentin Letts shows support for Wakefield when he describes Wakefield as:

> ..simply a good man who was troubled by the scientific evidence he found.
>
> (*Daily Mail* 4 February 2002)

Wakefield was labelled as 'no longer working' or 'forced out' of the Royal Free Hospital. Theoretically, this point could have been used to discredit Wakefield but in the vast majority of cases journalists did not frame his employment situation as such. Instead, this style of reporting framed Wakefield as being unfairly treated and that someone, somewhere was trying to cover up the truth (with the government most often accused).

Accusations of Inaccuracy

One of the most common outcries from scientists and health professionals about mainstream media coverage of their own research is 'that's inaccurate!' But is this a fair complaint? Many scientific and health stories originate from research published in peer-reviewed journals. Journalists are then required to reduce these lengthy and complex articles into 2-minute stories or 300-word articles aimed at the general public. The job of a journalist is not to only précis and simplify research, but also to explain its relevance and make it newsworthy. These last two points – relevance and newsworthiness – can mean scientific detail may be omitted or appear less prominently, thus affecting accuracy. The purpose of an academic peer-reviewed article is very different from the purpose of a story in the mainstream media. Scientists' concerns about accuracy in the mainstream media often fails to acknowledge this difference. Dornan warns that this concern about accuracy can have a significant impact on expectations of coverage; '(t)here is a slide from the premise that journalism should be required to get the scientific details right to the assertion that these details themselves dictate the form and tone that coverage should adopt' (1999: 185).

Numerous studies examine accuracy by comparing original scientific research to its media coverage. For example, Molitor (1993) examined the media's coverage of using aspirin to prevent heart attacks and criticised the media for inaccuracies in this coverage and for sensationalising the scientific research (for similar research see also Bell 1994, Singer 1990, Boyd-Barrett et al. 1977). Criticism of media inaccuracy relies on the idea that there is an objective truth in science, but this fails to acknowledge the tentative nature of scientific knowledge, as Karpf points out:

> The medical profession generally attributes crises to the media's inaccuracy, as if accuracy, objectivity and truth were unproblematic notions...At the heart of many crises in medico-journalist relations are medical disagreements, with the messenger as scapegoat.
>
> (1988: 168)

Arguments that put accuracy at the heart of analysing the quality of science or medical journalism, such as '(t)here is no neutral or objective way of communicating science, but truth and accuracy ought to be our guide' (Miller 1999: 224), fail to acknowledge the complexities of the terms 'accuracy' and 'truth'.

These accuracy studies, carried out primarily by social scientists, assume that scientists are concerned about accuracy, but when asked if they were troubled about accuracy in stories concerning their research, scientists expressed low levels of concern and instead were more interested in the story's wider context and presentation (Hansen and Dickinson 1992). Maier (2002) performed accuracy studies on a wide range of news sources and found a similar lack of concern about accuracy. He concluded that news sources were less concerned with factual errors than with more subjective or interpretive errors.

The content analysis of newspaper, television and radio coverage revealed concerns about accuracy in the coverage of the MMR/autism story are unfounded: few scientific facts were reported 'incorrectly'. Instead, as Hansen and Dickinson found, more subtle journalistic processes influenced the tone and context. As will be discussed in Chapter 4, balancing evidence and balancing sources unfairly reflected the level of scientific research supporting Wakefield.

The audience research also highlights the irrelevance of analysing accuracy in media coverage of science and health. Parents' decisions about the MMR vaccine had little to do with possessing high levels of accurate knowledge. As Chapter 8 will explore, parents did not remember the details of the story; in fact, many could not remember simple facts such as Wakefield's name, or details of his research. Focus groups remembered the broader message that the MMR vaccine might be linked to autism but failed to remember details of the coverage. This vague awareness that the MMR vaccine might be unsafe was what made parents sceptical of the MMR vaccine, not the details of Wakefield's research. Therefore, *even if* accuracy were found to be a problem in the content analysis, it is important to note the public did not remember specific details about complicated scientific debates and instead remembered broader themes.

Stating coverage is 'inaccurate' is too vague a complaint, and scientists and media researchers need more specific analyses when examining why coverage is problematic. Issues concerning certainty, narrative, controversies, balance and source selection all have a more substantial impact on how the media cover health, science and risk stories.

Binary Oppositions and Excessive Certainty

In the process of making issues less complex, journalists use a variety of journalistic practices, one of which is creating binary oppositions. This 'oppositional' style of reporting is a conventional method used by journalists to simplify complicated stories or to represent objectivity. Fursich and Lester (1996) analysed the *New York Times* science column and revealed how journalists constructed scientific work as either 'good' science or 'bad' science. Representations of contemporary mass media health are often framed in a 'series of core oppositions', for example, 'the dangers of modern life, villains and freaks; victimhood; professional heroes and lay heroes' (Seale 2004: 9).

In the coverage of the MMR/autism story it was not the division of scientific evidence into two camps that was the most significant binary opposition because the evidence was so one-sided. The vast majority of evidence demonstrates the MMR vaccine is the safest way to protect a child from measles, mumps and rubella. Instead, the most common binary opposition was to juxtapose the 'dangerous' MMR vaccine with the 'safer' single vaccines. Single jabs were frequently discussed—in 64% of all stories (68% in tabloids and down to 55% in the broadsheets), 79% of the TV news stories and 53% of the *Today* programme stories. The high appearance of single vaccines on television is attributed to journalists using single vaccine clinics as backdrops for pieces-to-camera; they offered an easy place to interview parents concerned about the MMR vaccine.

Single vaccines made even more of an impact in outlets which campaigned against the MMR jab. If we compare anti-MMR outlets with pro-MMR outlets, single vaccines were mentioned in 79% of *Daily Mail* articles, 71% of *The Sun*'s articles but only 40% of articles in *The Mirror*. Many editorials and news articles in the *Mail* and *Sun* emphasised the safety of the single vaccines over the MMR vaccine and paid a great deal of attention to the fact that single vaccines should be made available for free on the NHS but without making it clear why they were safer. Rarely did articles critically examine why single vaccines might be safer and instead stated single vaccines were *the* solution to the controversy. In the following *Sun* leader, they demand choice between the MMR and single vaccines, simply because their readers deserve this choice:

MMR SCANDAL: LACK OF CHOICE

THE arrogant people who run the NHS are refusing Sun readers a vital choice over the health of their children. They won't let YOU decide whether your child has the controversial MMR triple jab or three single ones...It is now clear that the lack of choice is a national scandal. Our readers' kids are at risk. Our readers simply have NO choice. OUR READERS ARE BEING TREATED LIKE SECOND CLASS CITIZENS.

(emphasis in article *The Sun* 5 February 2002)

That the media consistently juxtaposed coverage in terms of whether or not parents *should* have the choice between single jabs or the MMR vaccine is significant. Lewis points out the power of creating oppositions: 'If the informational media can influence opinion simply by talking about X rather than Y – without, apparently, needing to express a single opinion – then information itself is deeply implicated in the construction of political ideology' (2001: 102). Thus the media's tendency to reduce the debate to two choices to either the MMR vaccine or to abandon the triple jab in favour of safer, single vaccines led to parents assuming that the vaccines were safer if given individually, even though there was no evidence to suggest this was the case.

Linked to the process of making issues less complex by reducing a story to binary oppositions is presenting results or findings as more certain than they are and ignoring the inherent uncertainty of science. A familiar complaint from scientists and health professionals is that coverage is presented as 'too certain' or 'over-certain'. Journalists presented the safety of single vaccines as more certain than it was, most often failing to state the absence of evidence. Journalists used practices such as depending on anonymous, nebulous sources (often labelled 'critics') to claim the safety of single vaccines over the triple jab.

Doubts about MMR began when it was claimed there could be a link between the vaccine and autism. Critics said parents should be given the choice of having separate jabs against each of the diseases on the NHS instead of the combined vaccine.

(*News of the World* 10 February 2002)

In the case of MMR, journalists' deliberate efforts to make some issues more certain led to hyperbole. Journalist made the dangers of the outbreaks more certain, by repeatedly framing the measles outbreaks as 'a major public health emergency'. This was a deliberate exaggeration of facts in order to make the story more newsworthy, as the following front page opening paragraph demonstrates. (At this stage measles cases were limited to a small number of nurseries in London and North East England.)

> The government was last night struggling to avert a major public health emergency over dwindling public confidence in the safety of the MMR vaccine, despite Tony Blair's insistence that expert scientific opinion overwhelmingly backs the controversial triple jab.
>
> (*The Guardian* 7 February 2002)

Other journalists made the validity or strength of the link between autism and the MMR vaccine more certain, such as in statements like the following:

> THOUGH measles can be a killer, it is little wonder parents remain fearful over the triple MMR injection. Whatever the medical establishment claim, the FACT is that hundreds of toddlers have become victims of irreversible autism or bowel disease after the multiple jab.
>
> (emphasis in original, *News of the World* 3 February 2002)

It might be true that the toddler became ill after the MMR vaccine, but no evidence has yet to prove the MMR vaccine caused the illness, but statements such as above suggested otherwise. These linguistic practices made the link between autism and the MMR vaccine more certain. In another example, the link is made more certain by stating a child 'developed' autism, instead of this being reported as a parent's claim:

> FRANTIC Kay McDonagh is hoping to find the cash to give her second child single vaccinations — because her first developed autism after the triple jab.
>
> (*The Sun* 7 February 2002)

Another way journalists made the link more certain was to juxtapose the rise in autism with the introduction of the MMR vaccine.

> However, there is no consensus on the factors causing the increase, except that it may have gathered pace over the same period as the MMR jab was being introduced...Other countries have seen rises. Rates have tripled in some U.S. states since MMR was introduced.
>
> (*Daily Mail* 7 February 2002)

Not all journalists fell into the trap of making excessively hyperbolic statements, or reporting measles outbreaks as particularly meaningful. *ITV* science editor Lawrence McGinty follows a report from his news correspondent colleague about the rise in measles cases and appears to contradict what his colleague has just reported:

We need to keep a sense of perspective here. We have so far 7 confirmed cases, 4 in the north east three in south London. Now that compares with an average year in which you would get something like a hundred outbreaks of suspected measles across the country and perhaps 40, 50, 60 confirmed cases. So I don't think we're looking at anything abnormal and we're certainly not in the middle of an epidemic where the disease is spreading from place to place in the country.

(*ITV* News 5 February 2002)

Journalists not only presented the scientific evidence relating to the MMR and single vaccines as more certain, but many journalists also expected science itself to guarantee certainty. More often it was general news correspondents, or in the case of the *Today* programme, its anchors, demanding certainty from science. In the following excerpt, *Today* anchor John Humphries demands a level of certainty from Labour MP Stephen Ladyman (a former scientist).

Humphries: Can you be absolutely certain that the increase in the incidence of MMR over the past few years is totally unrelated to MMR? The increase in autism, I beg your pardon, is totally unrelated to MMR?
Ladyman: As a scientist myself you can never prove a negative and all I can say is that all the evidence points away from that being the correct hypothesis. All the evidence suggests that MMR is safe. The science that is, that links MMR to autism is, at best, circumstantial and is largely anecdotal and you can't base public health policy on that sort of information.

(*Today* BBC radio 14 February 2002)

On 3 February 2002 a tabloid editorial demanded a 100% guarantee that science simply cannot provide:

...he (Prime Minister) must produce the evidence that MMR is absolutely danger-free.

(*News of the World* 3 February 2002)

All of the above examples—stories which emphasised the dangers and extent of the outbreaks of measles as definite proof that parents were rejecting the MMR vaccine (when this was not the case), linguistic practices which made the link between the MMR vaccine and autism and journalists' failure to understand the tentative nature of science—demonstrate how certainty was problematic in the media coverage of the MMR/autism link.

Specialist and General News Correspondents

Alongside the increasing coverage of science and health in the Western media (see, for instance, Clayton et al. 1993, Hijmans et al. 2003, Entwistle and Beaulieu-Hancock 1992, Nelkin 1987) is an increase in specialist correspondents reporting science and health. However, the increase in science and health is so vast that specialists are not the only journalists who cover these stories. An examination of over 12,000 science and technology stories covering the first 6 months of 2004 and 2006 in 6 national newspapers (daily and Sunday), the late evening television news bulletins on BBC1 and ITV and the *Today* programme on Radio 4 found that only 10% of stories were covered by health and science specialists (Boyce et al. 2007). The function of specialist health and science correspondents is not to write or present *every* science and health story (indeed, political stories are written by many journalists and not just political correspondents), but one of their primary functions is to act as the key contact for medical and scientific journals and organisations and relevant government departments. Health and science journals and sources target specialist correspondents and direct their press releases to them. But for most of these sources, the established and good relationships they have with specialist correspondents are often irrelevant as most science and health stories are written by general news correspondents, as was the case in the MMR/autism story.

Health and science correspondents produced only a quarter of the MMR/autism stories in the sample with a significant variation between media outlets. Science/medical correspondents were more likely to present stories on television where they presented just under 40% of the stories. All stories on the *Today* programme in the sample period were presented by general news correspondents, and even though they do not appear, specialist correspondents on the *Today* programme provide briefings for anchors and still influence reports. Not only were most stories written by non-specialists, but there was a large number of journalists reporting the MMR/autism story. Eighty-one different news journalists appeared in the sample, suggesting this was a story that required little background knowledge or established contacts. Many sources interviewed referred to the problem of journalists 'dropping into' the story with little or no knowledge of the background of the debate. Those interviewed stated they were accustomed to dealing with journalists who knew little of the scientific details or background to the MMR/autism story.

> There are journalists who are new or whatever and come in and think this is a great debate and I guess the frustrating thing is…a lot of the research is not really new, it's actually recycled or you know, whatever, it's not actually brand new research. And I think the frustration is sometimes that journalists, particularly one who's not been on board the debate for the five plus years, doesn't actually know this actually isn't new. So you get headlines like 'Cutting edge research' or whatever saying 'x-y-z' and in fact it's a study that went on a year and a half ago.
>
> (Patients' group)

And many contrasted the coverage by generalists with the higher standard produced by specialists.

> Generally, we've not needed to work very hard with the health correspondents on broadcast news. I mean they know the science, they know the evidence and they try and present that evidence um pictorially. I remember seeing (BBC journalist) Fergus Walsh doing a piece just explaining what the balance of the evidence was in pictures, it was really fantastic and the same with…(ITV journalist) Lawrence McGinty I think he'd done stuff as well which was really quite, presenting the weight of evidence and showing that it's overwhelmingly in favour of MMR and against alternatives.
>
> (Health communication PR)

Most sources interviewed alleged *who* reported a story influenced *how* it was reported stating the general news correspondents were 'the problem'. The suspicions of the sources interviewed are correct: there were differences in the way specialists and generalists reported the MMR/autism story. Looking at how journalists led their stories, what they chose to emphasise to draw the audience in reveals a difference. Health and science correspondents used new research as a lead in 21% of their stories, compared to 13% for other journalists. In almost complete contrast, generalists used political statements in the lead of 24% of their stories compared to 15% for health and science correspondents. General news correspondents used the drama of personal experiences in the lead of 7% of their stories, whilst this did not occur once in stories written by health/science correspondents. Clearly generalists were more comfortable using politics or human interest to attract audiences.

There were also differences in the sources used by specialist health and science correspondents versus generalists. Both groups sourced politicians, scientists and health professionals and pressure groups in much the same way (making up 46% of sources used by science and health correspondents and 48% of sources used by all other journalists). The differences came when examining how parents and the Department of Health were sourced. Science and health correspondents, having established relationships with the DoH, were three times more likely to source them (22% of all sources versus 6%). Instead, generalists were more likely to turn to parents (15% versus 9%) and sourcing other journalists in the newsroom (7% versus 1%).

Looking at more specific uses of sources reveals more significant differences. Different journalists chose different sources to question the safety of the MMR vaccine or to state its safety; specialists were more likely to use scientists in both cases. In contrast, general news correspondents were more likely to use parents to *question* the MMR vaccine's safety and were more likely to use a range of sources to argue the MMR vaccine's safety, or, as occurred in a quarter of all stories, not include any information about the vaccine's safety (see Tables 2.1, 2.2). Using the claims of parents was a simple way to frame the story as these opinions were easy to find compared to locating relevant scientific expert-sources.

Table 2.1 How different journalists reported who questions MMR vaccine's safety

Source questioning safety	Health/Science Correspondents	General news journalists
Scientist/Health professional	36%	21%
Parent	21%	38%
Journalist (in article)	24%	12%
Politician	9%	8%
JABS or activists	7%	9%
Other	2%	4%
Wakefield	2%	4%
Journalist	0%	5%

Whilst different journalists used the same *types* of sources, they used the statements from sources in different ways, which gave more or less prominence and validity to different scientific arguments.

Analysing the sources selected by specialists is important, for one of the main criticisms made of specialists is that their relationships

Table 2.2 How different journalists reported who stated MMR vaccine's safety

Source stating safe	Health/Science Correspondents	General news journalists
Scientist	37%	32%
DoH/CMO/'health chiefs'	27%	19%
Not stated safe	14%	24%
Politician/ government	17%	14%
BMA, WHO, Royal Colleges, MRC, PHLS/HPA	5%	3%
Other	0%	6%
Reported by journalist	0%	2%
Parent	0%	1%

with sources are too familiar to remain 'objective' (Tunstall 1971, Dunwoody 1978, Crouse 1974, Ehrlich 1995). Nelkin is critical of this point and argues all journalists, when they report science stories, are more trusting of sources because:

> '(u)sually the reporter cannot assess the experience of these scientists, their knowledge of the subject, or their reliability as sources. Faced with technical terms that are difficult to check out, and socialised to regard scientists as a reliable and objective source of information, these journalists are inclined to believe what they are told'.
>
> (1995 in Levi 2001: 12)

Nelkin's point is important – journalists, whether specialists or not, depend on sources to explain complex scientific concepts/information. But this trusting relationship is less helpful when scientists disagree. Which scientists do journalists 'believe what they are told'?

Instead of the close relationship between sources and journalists, what is more relevant in the MMR/autism story is the accusation that specialists are influenced by the informal network which exists between them (Tunstall 1971, Zelizer 1997). One source, a former journalist, explained the impact of this network on the way stories are reported.

> If you come to a press conference with health correspondents…at the end of it there's a little knot of them gathered together afterwards and what they say is 'well what do you think the story is?' They discuss what they all think the story is and they go away and most of the time they all write exactly the same story cause they've discussed it. They're very frightened of being out on a limb and writing a completely different story to what *The Telegraph*, *The Mail* and *The Guardian* have got cause their news editor will say 'Hang on, they've all got that story why have you got something else?'
>
> (Health communication PR)

These were some similarities in the way generalist and specialist journalists reported the MMR/autism story. They both included similar information as shown in Table 2.3.

Table 2.3 How different journalists reported key messages in the MMR/autism story

Content	Health/Science correspondents	General news journalists*
Single vaccines	12%	12%
Vaccination levels dropping	10%	11%
Should be a choice in vaccines	10%	11%
MMR is safe	9%	8%
Measles outbreaks	7%	8%
Leo Blair	5%	6%
Private clinics	3%	6%
Government made mistakes in past and cannot be trusted	2%	2%

*This includes both general news correspondents and other specialists (such as political or economic specialists).

What are the implications of general news correspondents reporting specialist subjects? The knowledge, contexts and background information are not as detailed when health and science stories are covered by general news correspondents. Specialists and general news correspondents might have included much of the same information in their stories, but the two groups used sources to position their arguments in very different ways. As a result of the criticism the media have received, specialists now more frequently report the MMR/autism story:

In the last year (2003)...in terms of any major MMR stories, it's always the science or health correspondents. I've asked a few of them about this...and they have told me... they think the criticisms of their output, whether it's newspaper or broadcast, on the issue of GM and on MMR, the criticism was that by putting the political correspondents on it, who have not a clue about the science, they got it wrong, they had major inaccuracies. They think that has stung their editors.

(Science communication PR)

Peer Review

Many health and science stories in the mainstream media emanate from academic journals, thus any issue concerning the peer review system will have an impact on media coverage. Research appearing in any academic journal is peer-reviewed to assess the validity and reliability of its findings. This is normally a straightforward process: the journal editor appoints 2 or 3 academics who are familiar with the field of research and the academics produce a written report outlining their opinion on the research. The system is not a 100% guarantee that the research is not falsified or somehow problematic but it 'is good at weeding out claims that can be seen as inconsistent. But it is not so good at detecting claims that are plausible but incorrect' (Labinger 2001: 263). Peer review is the most efficient method which permits research to be published without having to repeat the experiment or research.

In very specialised fields like science and health that require knowledge of a wide range of topics, peer review has the important function to help journalists understand the significance and reliability of research. Journalists rely 'heavily on journal peer review processes and the opinions of medical experts to guide them in the selection and development of stories' (Entwistle 1995: 922). Even when the peer review process is under scrutiny, journalists still rely on it for they lack the expertise to discriminate between good and bad or questionable research.

In recent years, the reliability and trust in peer review in the sciences[3] has come under scrutiny because of a number of scandals.[4] The Hwang scandal has made the most serious dent in the confidence of peer review. Professor Hwang published research in the leading journal *Science* in 2004 claiming to be the first scientist to clone 30 human embryos and harvest stem cells from one of them. Hwang published further peer-reviewed research in May 2005 (again in *Science*) claiming to have established 11 stem-cell lines derived from the skin cells of individual patients. Even though both papers were fully peer-reviewed, allegations of unethical research arose in November 2005 followed by accusations of scientific fraud one month later. In a teary speech after these accusations were made public, Hwang admitted his stem cell research was fabricated and his papers about human cloning were subsequently withdrawn. Rob Stein, science reporter on the *Washington Post,* reflects on the impact the Hwang controversy and the manipulation of the peer review process on journalism:

> My antennae are definitely up since (Hwang controversy). I'm reading papers a lot more closely than I had in the past, just to sort of satisfy myself that any individual piece of research is valid. But we're still in sort of the same situation that the journal editors are, which is that if someone wants to completely fabricate data, it's hard to figure that out. (Bosman 2006)

In light of these scandals the science community has sought to reaffirm the public's trust in science. The Royal Society, a long-established independent academy promoting excellence in science in the UK, convened a working group to examine some of these issues. This group was initially asked to examine how the peer review process could be made more robust because of controversial research published by Hwang and Wakefield. However, in the case of the MMR/autism story, the peer review process was not where the problem lay – Wakefield's research was peer reviewed many times. The problem for the Royal Society was that Wakefield made his accusations outside of his peer-reviewed research, much to the frustration of the scientific community. Eventually the working group acknowledged that peer review was not the primary problem in the MMR/autism story and the Royal Society review then became more concerned with how scientific results were communicated to the public. The report concluded scientists should assess the potential impact of research results on the public and that it is *scientists'* responsibility to ensure these results are 'appropriately' communicated. They absolved the media of blame. The efforts to improve how science is communicated are welcome, but journalists do have a role in how science and health is communicated, especially when they report assertions that are not peer-reviewed. Wakefield made some of his most serious claims linking the MMR vaccine to autism in press conferences. These statements, far from being ignored, can have and did have, a significant impact as they were made directly to journalists.[5] For example, as outlined in Chapter 1, the idea that single vaccines are safer than the triple vaccine was first publicly suggested by Wake-field in the 1998 Royal Free press conference. Wakefield based this theory on the idea that the triple vaccine overloaded the immune sys-tem and therefore it was safer to give the vaccines separately[6] (he never made the claim that it was unsafe to give three vaccines simul-taneously in the Diphtheria-Tetanus-Pertussis vaccine). As explained, Wakefield's claim was never examined in scientific research so there was no peer review evidence to support this claim. In the coverage analysed, the lack of evidence supporting Wakefield's claim that the immune system could be overwhelmed was rarely discussed in the media. When this claim was covered, any reference to alleged re-search that supports the claim was vague or not discussed:

> But previous theories have suggested that the triple vaccine may 'overload' the body and let measles take hold in the intestines.
>
> (*Daily Mail* 6 February 2002)

> I AM persuaded that some youngsters may react to MMR if their immune system is lowered.
>
> (Health editor Jackie Thorton *The Sun* 5 February 2002)

> It was February 1998 when Wakefield finally told a press conference at the Royal Free his study of 12 children with an unusual bowel syndrome had discovered traces of the measles virus in their guts. His working hypothesis was that the MMR jab might have damaged their immune systems, letting the virus take hold and leading somehow to the development of autism in some of the group.
>
> (*Observer* 10 February 2002)

Wakefield's claims about the dangers of the MMR vaccine were fur-ther amplified because other scientists were reluctant to comment on these non-peer-reviewed claims, believing they were not worth com-ment because the evidence had not been through the peer review process. Therefore Wakefield's non-peer-reviewed claims often went unchallenged, or when scientists did respond, they did so in vague and general terms, as they were unsure of exactly what to respond to. One of the specialist correspondents interviewed was aware of this problem.

> If you are presented with a new paper or piece of evidence from Wakefield that nobody else has seen yet, they will say to you "well, it's very difficult to comment because I haven't seen it but in general there is this, this and this". The story will probably be Andrew Wakefield comes up with new piece of evidence that he claims says this but everybody else says probably wrong

because of this but they can't say for sure because they haven't seen the evidence, it's as simple as that really.

(Health editor)

Other journalists viewed Wakefield's attempts to secure coverage in the mainstream media by avoiding the peer-review process as understandable.

> He's behaving in an unorthodox way for a scientist, but then he's not got a conventional message so you probably wouldn't expect him to be a conventional scientist about it. The dissidents have to behave in a different way...I suppose he will do whatever he can to try to get people to take notice of what he's saying.

(Health editor)

Medical journals have admitted they played a role in sustaining coverage of the MMR vaccine when they chose to publish Wakefield's research. By 2002 few prestigious journals published Wakefield's work and instead he depended on smaller journals.[7] Editors of medical journals who published Wakefield's research were aware the publication might give publicity to Wakefield's theories and thus affect the MMR uptake rates and sought to control this influence by publishing related editorials. An editorial accompanied the original 1998 *Lancet* article written by two scientists from the Centers for Disease Control and Prevention in the USA. This editorial argued Wakefield's findings should be considered in light of the millions of people who have received measles-containing vaccines since the 1960s and had no adverse reaction. It concluded that Wakefield's research 'may snowball into societal tragedies when the media and the public confuse association with causality and shun immunisation' (Chen and Stefano 1998: 611). Another editorial accompanied Wakefield and Montgomery's 1999 publication in the *Israeli Medical Association Journal* stating '(t)he evidence that MMR is implicated in either Crohn's disease or autism is flimsy at best, and until more definitive evidence and further insights are obtained, the medical community should strongly resist any change in the present vaccination policy' (Passwell 1999: 177). When *Molecular Pathology* carried Wakefield's February 2002 article it also had an editorial that warned: 'in no way can the data presented here be used to support the generalisation that MMR causes all autism and/or inflammatory diseases of the bowel' (Morris and Aldulaimi 2002). But these editorials had little influence on the subsequent coverage and served only to rebuff accusations that journals published Wakefield's research only to attract attention.

The editor of *The Lancet,* Richard Horton, has consistently defended his decision to publish Wakefield's 1998 paper, arguing that it had successfully passed through the normal peer-review process and any problems with the findings or conclusions would have been picked up at this stage.[8] Horton remained unrepentant about his decision to publish Wakefield's article until Brian Deer's research surfaced in 2004. It was only after the revelations of a conflict of interest in February 2004 that Horton admitted that '(t)he story was by *now* political, not medical' (emphasis added, 2004a: 7). He goes on to state that in 2004 '(j)ournalists *now* began to personalise as well as to politicise the storm...Liam Donaldson...proceeded to wade into a *now* wholly confused debate accusing Wakefield of doing "poor science"' (emphasis added, 2004a: 8). Horton declared that the story was political in 2004, even though the non-medical media had consistently covered the story since 1998, with periods of significant interest. Certain news outlets like the *Daily Mail,* the *Evening Standard* and *Private Eye* were selectively publishing MMR stories primarily supportive of Wakefield's work and the views of JABS parents. Why Horton did not view this coverage as political is unclear.

The lack of peer review behind a scientific proposition would not necessarily mean journalists would avoid publishing the claim, for, ultimately, a newsworthy story is more important than one that is scientifically sound. Journalists can make it clear in an article that the claim is not peer-reviewed, but still give it prominent coverage.

> If things were not in peer reviewed journals then I'd kind of want to know why...That's not to say that we would never not write a story because it was not in a peer reviewed journal. But if I was doing that I'd make it extremely clear the provenance, without libelling people obviously! (laughs)
>
> (Health editor)

For example, months after the flurry of front page articles about the MMR/autism story in February 2002, the *Today* programme reported on research not yet peer-reviewed. Openly stating the research was not peer-reviewed or published, they nonetheless spent more than 10 minutes discussing the research:

> Now one of the researchers who's involved in work on the MMR jab is claiming that he's found reason to suspect that some cases of autism could be related to the triple jab. Paul Shattock is director of the Autism Research Unit at the University of Sunderland. His work has not yet been peer reviewed, subjected to scrutiny by other scientists, through peer review, it hasn't been fully published yet. But he does say that a study of 4000 cases of

autism in this country suggests to him that around 10 of them could have
been triggered by some reaction to the MMR jab.

(*Today* BBC radio 27 June 2002)

The peer review process is not a 100% guarantee that science is valid,
but it is the best method to date that can distinguish and discriminate
between claims. When scientists make unsubstantiated claims, without research to support it and seek to get media coverage, this un-
dermines the peer review process and ultimately alters trust in
scientists and the scientific process.

The BSE Effect

Since the 1990s the Bovine Spongiform Encephalopathy (BSE) crisis
has been the most influential science and health story in the UK and it
continues to have a substantial impact. The UK Ministry of Agriculture, Fisheries and Food first discussed publicly the discovery of BSE
in animals in 1987. Two years later, in 1989, the UK government made
its first statement that there was no risk of BSE to humans and that
eating beef was safe. Over the next seven years the UK government
either maintained this line or remained fairly silent on the issue (see
Kitzinger and Reilly 1997 for a comprehensive assessment of the media's coverage of the BSE crisis). The government was acting on its
best scientific advice as well as desperately trying to halt the decline
in UK beef sales. In a gesture to publicly verify the safety of British
beef, Conservative MP and Minister of Agriculture John Gummer in-
famously fed his young daughter a beef burger in 1990. After a dec-
ade of denying BSE was a risk to humans, in 1996 the Conservative
government announced 10 people had died from a new form of
Creutzfeldt-Jacob Disease (CJD), caused by eating BSE-infected meat.
In the 1990s scientist Dr. Richard Lacey was one of the very few
voices warning BSE might be fatal to humans. Lacey accused the government and scientists of a "systematic cover-up" about the dangers in
the food Britons eat but Lacey and other proponents of the BSE/CJD
link were maligned and silenced. His repeated efforts to attract media
attention to the issue soon bored journalists, who viewed him as a
maverick seeking attention, as the following journalist states.

One of the most devastating things a news desk can ever say to a journalist
is: 'I think we know that, don't we?' in a very sarcastic voice. So it wouldn't
have done me any good to wander up and say 'Oh, Professor Lacey is still

very worried that we might all get some weird brain disease from moo cows'. The news desk would say 'sod off, we know that, he's said it before'.

(Kitzinger and Reilly 1997: 343)

Journalists dismissed him, but as history has shown, Lacey was correct.

The BSE crisis was not frequently directly discussed in the media coverage of the MMR/autism story. Comparisons with previous scientific controversies appeared in only 13% of stories, with the BSE/CJD crisis the most common comparison (the Genetically Modified (GM) food and foot-and-mouth crises were less common comparisons). It was in interviews that journalists revealed the impact of the BSE crisis on the way they reported the MMR/autism story. They were anxious not to be caught out again, as they believed they were on BSE, by elevating government opinion over a single scientific source or by ignoring the views of a 'maverick' scientist. This view only occasionally appeared in the media coverage.

> The unconfirmed findings of maverick scientists such as Dr Andrew Wakefield prey upon a public which has grown at once more consumerist and more sceptical of authority, with good reason after the BSE and foot and mouth fiascos.
>
> (*The Observer* 10 February 2002)

In an overview of the BSE controversy, Agony Aunt[9] Dr. Miriam Stoppard blames previous science scandals and the government's role in these as reasons for the public's scepticism.

> ...I studied Dr Wakefield's paper and was horrified to see the conclusions he had drawn from sloppy research. However, I'm not surprised that his statements have been taken up by parents and the media alike. The public has grown sceptical of authority and scientists and who can blame them — thalidomide, salmonella, BSE and foot and mouth. ...Is there a part of intelligent people that science just can't reach? Is there impenetrable scepticism about science? Are scientists — and health educators — seen as untrustworthy? And if so, how do we alter that?
>
> (*The Mirror* 14 February 2002)

Even though it was not frequently directly referred to in media coverage, it was apparent in interviews with both sources and journalists that BSE was a frame used by journalists and sources when deciding how to report the story. Framing analysis more commonly analyses media content and media coverage would suggest BSE was irrelevant, but the production analysis in the MMR/autism story reveals the powerful frame the BSE crisis had over this story. With the BSE/CJD controversy not long from the top of the news agenda, journalists were quick to view the MMR/autism story as the next possible government cover-up, or 'BSE Part Two'. The following demonstrates the extent to which BSE acts as a frame for future health and science stories that involve the government and science.

> (The MMR/autism story) very quickly became not about good science versus bad science, whether the MMR was safe or not from the media point of view; it was *BSE Part Two*. Here was an anti-establishment scientist saying something and you got these government scientists being rolled out saying 'it's absolutely safe'. And the news editors and news desks had seen it before.
>
> (Science editor)

In interviews, journalists repeatedly stated they regarded this story as 'the next' controversial science story. Their experience in reporting the BSE crisis led them to suspect a government or science conspiracy:

> When one of the white coats starts to metaphorically beat the other white coat round the head is where the media takes great interest…partly because we might smell a rat. I smelt a rat very early in this case because the Department of Health was frankly beating poor old Wakefield metaphorically round the head.
>
> (Science editor)

The possibility that Wakefield might be the next Lacey also figured significantly in sources' minds. When the government or science made statements about 'trusting the evidence' of the MMR vaccine's safety, both sources and journalists were aware the public would not be so quick to trust this information.

> I know that post-BSE, post-GM there is a sense that the government saying "This is safe" can no longer be trusted. We've all got the image of John Gummer eating his beef burger (laughs), that's one thing that I'm sure played into it.
>
> (Science communication PR)

> Nobody trusts the medical establishment totally; less and less in these days than perhaps they did once.
>
> (Health editor)

Both sources and journalists continue to regard the BSE crisis as an influential frame in the reporting of science and health. Scientific and government statements about the safety of the MMR vaccine were thus received with scepticism and suspicion. The BSE crisis, now more than 10 years old, continues to have considerable influence on how science and health stories are reported in the UK.

The common criticisms made about health and science coverage—the tendency to make stories controversial, accurate, creating binary oppositions and reporting facts as 'certain'—had fluctuating relevance to the MMR/autism story. The story was undoubtedly a controversy in the UK, and how this controversy was created and sustained is examined further in the following chapter on news values. Accuracy was not identified as a problem, but the reduction of this complex story to two binary messages 'MMR is safe' versus 'MMR is not safe' was evident. Instead of obvious accuracy errors, coverage was problematic because of more subtle factors – including the way certainty was manufactured and the way Wakefield's claims, often made outside peer-reviewed journals, were reported as credible or valid. Part of the reason why scientific facts were occasionally disregarded (or made a low priority in the story) was because of the lasting impact of BSE on how science and health is reported in the UK. The following chapter further examines how many of these issues (controversy, trust, risks) influence which science and health stories are reported through an examination of news values.

CHAPTER THREE

News Values and Health, Science and Risk Stories

Research into the news values of stories emanates from media studies scholars' attempts to systematise why journalists select some stories over others. The first discussion of news values was Galtung and Ruge's 'The Structure of Foreign News' (1981). Their work, published more than 40 years ago, analysed a selection of crisis stories in foreign news and resulted in 12 categories of news values now widely used: frequency, threshold, unambiguity, meaningfulness, consonance, unexpectedness, continuity, composition, reference to elite nations, references to elite people, reference to persons and reference to something negative (Galtung and Ruge 1981: 12). They argued the more news values an event adheres to the more likely it is to be covered. Further, the news values which made the event initially newsworthy continue to influence the story's angle.

Harcup and O'Neill updated Galtung and Ruge's theory and also used newspapers to collate their list of news values. They analysed page leads in three national UK newspapers, and their contemporary set of news values are: the power elite, celebrity, entertainment, surprise, bad news, good news, magnitude (impact on numbers of people or potential impact), relevance, follow-up and newspaper agenda (2001: 279).

Using Galtung and Ruge's categories, the news values associated with MMR/autism story are: unambiguity (although the research linking the MMR vaccine and autism is ambiguous, the way the link was publicised and understood by the audience was unambiguous); continuity; reference to persons; and negativity. In Harcup and O'Neill's research, the MMR/autism story meets the following categories: surprise (a vaccine regarded as safe is suddenly not deemed safe); bad news; magnitude (most people have a connection to children – either as parents or through family or social relationships); relevance (vaccination is an enduring public health policy); follow-up (this story had 'legs' because of the constant stream of new research and parents claiming their children were affected); and newspaper agendas (although it is more appropriate to label this as *media* agendas). Neither of these lists provides adequate explanation as to why this story received such significant coverage compared to other science and health issues nor why it has continued to receive such substantial coverage.

These lists are useful in understanding which news is reported, but other factors affect what becomes news. There are periods when certain stories are more 'valuable' than at other times (Manning 2001: 61). For example, topics become more valuable simply because they already appear in the news; 'once a subject gains a certain news momentum it attracts more, and journalistic interest feeds on itself' (Kitzinger and Reilly 1997: 334, see also Cunningham 2003).

Beginning with a brief explanation of the evolution of news values, this chapter considers the particular news values in science, health and risk stories. Unlike Galtung and Ruge or Harcup and O'Neill, this analysis of news values examines the production, content and reception of a story to determine its values. It is also more comprehensive then Galtung and Ruge or Harcup and O'Neill as it considers television, radio *and* newspapers. Four specific news values are identified as to why certain health and science stories receive coverage when others do not.

- *Controversy.* If a health/science/risk story can be reported and framed as a controversy it is more likely to be covered. Using the rise in autism and the argument for single vaccines on the NHS, journalists were able to frame the MMR/autism story as controversial.
- *Editorial campaigns and pack journalism.* If a science or health story is attached to an editorial stance or a campaign, then its news values are increased. Certain media outlets used the MMR/autism story to make accusations about the NHS and the Labour government and then other media followed.
- *Framing health and science stories as political, not scientific.* If journalists are able to report without scientific detail or evidence, then the story is more attractive. In this case, journalists seldom

used research or evidence and instead chose to frame the story as more political than scientific.

- *Risk, trust and blame.* If a health and science story is about risk, trust or blame, or can be framed as such, then it has more news values. The MMR/autism story was frequently framed as a risk story and highlighted issues about risk and trust in modern society.

Research has yet to consider the specific news values of science and health stories. The idea that science news which is 'fascinating' or 'amazing' receives coverage (Resenberger 1997) is a common assumption; however, these words are merely synonyms for 'interesting'. What news values seek to do is identify what *is* interesting. The more relevant question is to understand why some stories are deemed 'fascinating' enough to receive media coverage. The need to make, what can be, esoteric subjects into something relevant to wider audiences is a key news value in the reporting of science and health: '(t)he most pronounced criterion of newsworthiness is whether science can be made recognisable to the reader in terms of human interest or in terms of something readers can relate to' (Hansen 1994: 114).

Farmelo argues scientists and journalists have different concepts of newsworthiness because scientists 'lack media savvy'. He highlights the 'cultural clash between science, in which accuracy, and peer review are treasured traditions, and the media, in which entertainment and contemporaneity are key virtues' (1997: 188). This clash is portrayed best in the coverage of controversies, for many health and science stories and sources are newsworthy because they are controversial or at least framed as controversial. This is particularly the case in science and health stories, yet 'controversy' does not appear in previous lists of news values.

Controversy

Journalists regularly use frames to simplify complex stories with the result that certain frames are chosen more often than others (Tuchman 1972). In the case of contemporary science and health stories, journalists create controversies or frame stories as controversial to make complex stories newsworthy. The media analysis reflected the findings from interviews with journalists and sources and the audience research; controversy was the most prominent news value. Many sources were former journalists and had years of experience working with the national media and were aware that journalists were likely to frame the MMR/autism story as a controversy. These sources knew that the appearance of a disagreement about a childhood vaccine and the resulting controversy would make a 'good' newsworthy story.

> It has all the ingredients for a science scare story/cause celebre in that you have a grain of truth in the fact there is scientific controversy. You have a science apparently split, you have the perception that someone is being unfairly treated for their maverick views.
>
> (MP)

Journalists who covered the story from its beginning identified the 1998 press conference held at the Royal Free Hospital as responsible for setting the initial controversial frame. At this press conference the public disagreement between Professor Arie Zuckerman, the dean of the hospital's medical school, and Dr. Andrew Wakefield provided journalists with an obvious frame:

> Professor Zuckerman...was urging everybody there very strongly, to be very cautious about the way they wrote the story. So he was there on the one hand playing it down if you like and Andrew Wakefield was there on the other side, *under his authority*, saying, "Look I've got this dramatic stuff to tell you!"....I think all the problems stem from that, come right from the start...it was very dramatic.
>
> (Health editor)

This press conference, and the way the scientific establishment responded, set the tone for how the story was reported in subsequent years. Journalists framed Wakefield as the next scientist exposing the hypocrisy of establishment (government) science. In 2004 all co-authors of the original 1998 *Lancet* paper, except Wakefield and one other scientist, disassociated themselves (again) from Wakefield's findings and his endorsement of single vaccines (Murch et al. 2004).[1]

One way journalists emphasised controversial news values in the MMR/autism story was to reduce the variety of scientific sources challenging Wakefield's theories to one homogeneous body. In doing so, they were then able to dismiss pro-MMR sources by labelling them as simply supporting the 'government'.

> There's the danger of anybody, if anybody speaks out supporting MMR as just being seen as a government spokesperson.
>
> (Health communication PR)

Sources argued that the MMR/autism story was being reported as the next scientific controversy and that the controversial frame added news value to the story. They claimed that because their official line of promoting the MMR vaccine was the same as the government's, they were then less newsworthy than those sources who continued to propagate the controversy.

> I think that (journalists) very much don't necessarily want to listen to what we have to say...They don't come to us anyway because we're not giving them what they want. They'd go to an organisation like JABS because obviously JABS are going to say much more controversial things than we are.
>
> (Patients' group)

These pro-MMR sources were aware their influence was limited because their views contained few news values and they were thus not amplifying the controversy.

Another way in which journalists found controversy in the MMR/autism story was by repeating Wakefield's claim that there was a conspiracy of scientists and government bureaucrats scheming against him. Wakefield and his supporters claimed that the government, other scientists and hospitals were deliberately silencing him but failed to provide proof of this, and by emphasising this claim, the story was made more newsworthy.[2]

> Ever since we first raised concerns about the MMR in '94 and Dr. Wakefield published his report what's been so worrying is the government and health chiefs have consistently refused to undertake meaningful research and have criticised any researcher that's presented them. They tried to make out that Dr Wakefield was a lone maverick when he's actually one of 12 researchers.
>
> (Jackie Fletcher, JABS spokesperson, *Today* BBC radio 17 June 2002)

Wakefield might have been 'one of 12 researchers' (and most of them eventually distanced themselves from Wakefield), but against this small group was the rest of the scientific community and published evidence.

A key principle for journalists is to be professional sceptics, to distrust what sources are telling them. In the case of the MMR/autism story, they believed that the best position was to be sceptical of the Labour government, but ultimately, this meant they were then giving a voice to a scientist who was making claims without any published or peer-reviewed evidence. In this case, scepticism was a naïve and ill-thought-out approach. Reed argues '(f)or journalists a major issue related to their sense of professionalism is the "right of dissenting groups from the mainstream to have a voice'" (2001: 290). In the case of the MMR/autism story, many journalists believed that publishing the views of dissenting scientists, and thereby exacerbating the controversy, was more newsworthy and fulfilled their role as sceptics. Inherent in scientific controversies is the question as to who has a right to comment and which views are relevant. As scientists argue amongst themselves, into this confusion steps journalists looking for newsworthy stories.

By far the most common way stories contained controversial news values was when they emphasised the link to autism rather than inflammatory bowel disease. In interviews journalists identified the link to autism and the associated controversy over the lack of known causes of autism, as the main reason why the story received such significant attention. (Cases of autism have increased since the 1970s and there is still no known cause.[3]) When asked why the story has consistently returned to the news agenda over five years many journalists were quick to state:

> Because there isn't an answer to autism…If there was more research into autism and they did find some sort of causal link then I think it would die down.
>
> (Health editor)

Instead of discussing the link between the MMR vaccine and inflammatory bowel syndrome or the general discussion that the MMR was unsafe, the media were emphasising the dangers of autism in order to attract the attention of worried parents. The media frequently reported the link between autism and the MMR vaccine; it appeared in over three-quarters (78%) of all stories in the period studied (see Figure 2.1 in Chapter 2, page 21) and in 10% of headlines. Again, the differences between media are striking. The *Mail on Sunday* mentions autism in all of its stories and the link is referred to in 93% of stories in the *Daily Mail*. Outlets which were not so obviously anti-MMR discussed autism less. The link appears in 67% of *BBC* news stories and 63% in *The Mirror*. Journalists who were also parents openly discussed their own worries about autism. One journalist spent most of her interview discussing autism and its effects on family life.

> I think that some of this outcry may be misplaced…but I think this is where the government should perhaps understand where some of this is coming from. Instead of just saying you've got to have this injection, it is safe. You have to understand the anxieties that are there. You go into any school now, any primary school and you've got this range of behavioural disorders,

some verging on the autistic spectrum that everybody knows about, whether they're working, middle-class I don't care. People are suddenly kind of afraid of this range of disorders now... I think the difficulty for lay people, such as myself, is to understand, is this rise in autism simply the result of better diagnosis?

(Newspaper columnist)

Many sources agreed that the reason why the story was newsworthy to journalists and the audience was the link to autism.

I think it's just that people are becoming more aware about autism. I mean autism is a very big issue, isn't it?

(Health communication PR)

But one journalist was frustrated that so much of the coverage concerned autism because it reinforced the idea that the link was real.

If you're doing a case history about someone with diabetes to show how difficult it is to be a diabetic and you know how you've got to inject yourself every morning and it's a pain and it hurts do you know what I mean? Then that's fair enough because what you're seeing on screen with the patient who is ill is directly relevant to the point you're trying to make, that diabetes is a horrible disease to have. With autism and MMR it's not. You see an autistic kid on the screen—that's not directly relevant to the MMR vaccine if the hypothesis is wrong, if Wakefield's hypothesis is wrong you're naturally sympathetic to that family. Then you have a parent who's said 'and in my opinion it was all after, shortly after we had the MMR vaccine'—now I think that conflates the two things.

(Science editor)

Few stories refer to current research examining the causes of autism and few covered Liam Donaldson's statements about autism given in a press conference in early February 2002 when he was promoting the MMR vaccine. *The Guardian's* health editor Sarah Boseley was the only journalist to cover Donaldson's statements on autism.

Autism is a complex range of conditions which manifest largely in behavioural problems. Genetic factors are thought to be important—as many as 10 genes might be involved, Prof Donaldson said. Most cases—70%—were in boys, yet boys and girls were equally represented in those receiving the MMR. He said that there had been a four-fold increase in autism in Britain between 1988 and 1993, and yet MMR vaccination rates had remained constant.

(*The Guardian* 8 February 2002)

During the sample period, autism received little coverage that did not also mention the MMR vaccine. In addition, for a story about autism and the MMR vaccine, very few experts on autism were sourced. When the *Daily Telegraph* surveyed autism experts from around the world they found 92% of the 52 experts polled found Wakefield's hypothesis extremely unlikely. But even the *Telegraph* did not let this evidence stand on its own and found a familiar anti-MMR scientist and supporter of Andrew Wakefield to challenge the autism experts:

> But Dr Paul Shattock, the head of autism research at Sunderland University, said: "I see teachers and psychologists who have no doubt that there is an increase. If you ask the Cambridge-London university axis then they would say no. But if you asked the people who have to get their hands dirty, you will get a different answer."
>
> *(Daily Telegraph* 6 September 2002)

The National Autistic Society (NAS) rarely appeared in the coverage and journalists did not mention the NAS in their interviews. When asked, journalists stated the NAS was not relevant.

> I rarely talk to them (NAS)...I don't think they've got any relevance to it cause I don't think it (MMR vaccine) causes autism.
>
> (Popular health editor)

There was intense disagreement within the National Autistic Society between those parents who believed there was a link between the disorder and the MMR vaccine and those who did not. This disagreement resulted in the NAS, for the most part, deliberately staying out of this debate. An opportunity to get out more information to parents interested in autism and its causes was thus missed. Journalists did not turn to relevant autism sources because, as will be discussed later, many of the journalists interviewed did not believe Wakefield's theory (Dearing 1994 also found that many journalists who report 'maverick' scientists do not believe in their theories). They used autism as a hook to interest their audience but their interest in autism stopped there.

Editorial Agendas and Pack Journalism

A story can have news values based on more than just the facts of the story itself (Harcup and O'Neill 2001). If a media outlet chooses to campaign on an issue, they can make any story newsworthy. Sources from both the pro- and anti-MMR side pointed to individual editors and owners using their newspapers to publicise their own concerns over the MMR/autism link.

> Quite often you will find that the editor's wife or the editor's aunt or the editor's somebody has suffered from something, that they want the newspaper to focus on Alzheimer's because their father just died, and so you do find this, this personal impact on something.
>
> (Health communication PR)

> Even though science correspondents were saying the weight of evidence is that there is no link between MMR and autism, editors were saying well yes, but you know, I've got an autistic daughter or my friend's got an autistic daughter and I think we really should be doing this story and asking questions and all that.
>
> (Health communication PR)

Many journalists referred to *The Sun*'s (weak) anti-MMR position, alleging that a single executive from its owners, News International, had a child with autism and believed this was linked to the MMR vaccine.

> If you have executives in the newspaper who know of someone who has an autistic child it plays much stronger with them than in an editorial brief where there isn't somebody with that experience.
>
> (Freelance science journalist)

In the UK, newspapers choose to adhere to political allegiances and they report stories through this filter. Radio and television journalists maintain they report in an objective and impartial manner[4]; for BBC journalists, presenting information 'objectively' and in a 'balanced' way is mandatory. When examining the output of campaigning news outlets like the *Daily Mail* and its sister paper the *Mail on Sunday* it is apparent that their political stance very much affected how the story was told by these two newspapers. The two papers framed the MMR/autism story as a reason to distrust the Labour government and a journalist working for one of these newspapers said the papers:

> ...us(ed) that (MMR vaccine) very much to attack the Prime Minister and the government personally...I don't think (the editors) would've particularly had a strong line on MMR had it not been for this.
>
> (Newspaper columnist)

The *Daily Mail* was particularly disparaging of the government in the coverage of the MMR/autism story. The language used in the following story demonstrates how the *Mail*'s coverage contributed to the idea that the government might be hiding something.

> He (CMO Dr. Liam Donaldson) spoke out as the *full might* of the medical establishment was *wheeled out* in a *desperate* bid to win back public confidence in the *controversy* over the combined vaccination.
>
> (emphasis added, *Daily Mail* 8 February 2002)

The Prime Minister's failure to disclose his son Leo's vaccination status gave already established anti-Labour media outlets a great opportunity to attack the government, and many journalists referred to the actions and influence of the right-wing media.

> They're (*Daily Mail*) sort of rabid dogs and you know they got hold of the whole thing of Leo not having it and they were using that very much to attack the Prime Minister and the government personally. But that attack could only have worked because this distrust was already there and this whole feeling you-do-as-we-say-not-as-we-do.
>
> (Newspaper columnist)

Sources also claimed that on occasion, one journalist in one media outlet could have a significant impact, as a journalist could pursue the MMR/autism story 'with a personal vendetta'. Many sources argued John Humphries of the BBC *Today* programme had a significant impact.

> I'd say the *Today* programme prevaricates depending on how John Humphries is feeling. It's true, cause he's got a small child now hasn't he? So the most recent one (interview with one of their members) he was incredibly anti (MMR)…he was extremely aggressive about the lack of choice but then you don't know whether if that's because of what's going on with the Hutton inquiry[5] and the BBC and the government being drawn into all of that. So he's very angry with the government.
>
> (Royal College)

When media outlets chose to campaign for or against an issue, in Britain's politically divided newspaper market, it is expected that outlets choose sides, as they did in the MMR/autism story. The left-leaning papers were more sympathetic to the Labour government's position, and some campaigned for the MMR vaccine, with one source laughing at *The Mirror*'s position.

> The popular press does tend to go one way or the other, I think it was *The Mirror* who phoned and said to me 'it's ok, *The Mirror* is pro-MMR', you

know they were very pro-MMR and that was going to be the line they were
going to take (laughing) — now they knew in advance they were pro-MMR!

(Royal College)

Media outlets who campaigned on this issue affected which scientific
research was deemed newsworthy. The reporting of scientific research was influenced by editorial agendas in the MMR/autism story.
On 6 February 2002 Wakefield published research in *Molecular Pathology*. This research was reported very differently in newspapers campaigning for and against the vaccine. The *Daily Mail* splashed the
research on its front page with the headline 'NEW ALERT ON MMR
JAB' with the following opening paragraph in an 858-word article:

> NEW research fuelled controversy over the MMR jab yesterday as fears
> grew of a large-scale measles outbreak. Scientists have for the first time es-
> tablished a possible link between the measles virus, autism and a related
> bowel disorder. The findings were revealed as clusters of measles, which can
> be fatal, emerged in London and the North-East.
>
> (*Daily Mail* 6 February 2002)

In contrast, *The Mirror*'s coverage appears on page eight and largely
covers the latest measles cases, with quotes supporting the safety of
the MMR from a health authority spokesperson, the DoH and a parent doubting the safety of their statements. The only reference to the
research is at the end of the 376-word article:

> The Department of Health said yesterday: "MMR is the safest and most ef-
> fective way of protecting children against measles, mumps and rubella."
> SCIENTISTS at Dublin University last night said they had found a possible
> link between measles and bowel disease and autism but advised people not
> to jump to conclusions.
>
> (capitals in original, *The Mirror* 6 February 2002)

The government's volte-face—arguing choice should be available
within the NHS but also stating that choice between the MMR and
single vaccinations was unwarranted—provided anti-Labour newspapers with an angle to pursue their editorial agenda and therefore
make it newsworthy. That single vaccines were not being provided on
the NHS was a way to criticise the Labour government's credibility.

> At a time when people were saying you have a choice in health care, here
> was something on which they could not have choice. That irked people be-
> cause they suddenly wanted to assert their rights as consumers when no-
> body had actually explained to them that actually, in this particular

incidence, asserting your rights means probably taking away the rights of another to remain healthy.

(Science journalist)

Journalists framed the Labour government as hypocritical, stating it sometimes supports choice in health care, but in the case of the MMR vaccine, it did not. The following editorial is typical of the accusations made against the government and shows how right-wing papers used the MMR/autism story to make wider political points:

> People now expect to enjoy choice in every other sphere of life, and well-informed but anxious mothers do not take kindly to suggestions of hysteria from their doctors—let alone from politicians. The MMR debate illustrates the more general problem faced by a centralised, tax-funded, state-controlled National Health Service in a prosperous, undeferential society.
>
> (*Daily Telegraph* 7 February 2002)

The Sun openly argued that paying for choice via private health care was not fair, because the high cost of single vaccines was not a choice for its less wealthy readers:

> Our readers' kids are at risk. Our readers simply have no choice. Our readers are being treated like second-class citizens.
>
> (*The Sun* 5 February 2002)

More than journalists or the audience, sources were frustrated with the contradiction of the government's commitment to offer choice in health care but then failing to offer choice between the MMR and single vaccines.

> It went to the heart of this whole business of choice and freedom which is a big political issue and I think the powerful mix of choice, freedom and big brother.
>
> (Health communication PR)

Sources argued journalists were correct to take the opportunity to challenge the government on their incongruous policy about choice in health care. They had little sympathy for the predicament the government had got themselves into.

> One thing I will definitely say is the government was hoist on their own petard...if they're offering choice then they can't turn around and deny it. That's one thing I hope the government has learnt.
>
> (Science communication PR)

Newspapers were not the only media outlets using the MMR/autism story to confront the government's contradictory position on choice in health care and purse an editorial agenda. Some sources also referred to the BBC *Today* programme's coverage and its editor at that time, Rod Liddle:

> It's now an open story—that Rod Liddle announced to everybody on the *Today* programme 'I believe there is a connection between MMR and autism and you will cover the story with that in mind'. So it was a direct instruction from Rod Liddle…I've been told by the majority of people, he, Rod Liddle, suggested that was really to subject the government to pressure and he thought this issue is fantastic. If you look at some of the papers that went for it, like the *Mail*, what do they most love? Having a go at the government, so it was definitely seen by the media as a great issue for them. And especially when the whole Leo Blair thing came in.
>
> (Science communication PR)

Scientists certainly believed that the media 'encouraged the campaign for single vaccines, which has been presented as an issue of choice and rights – and was taken up in these terms by opposition politicians' (Fitzpatrick 2002).

In the UK, the idea of choice in health care dominates health policy (see Pollock 2004) and this turn to 'choice' is seen in coverage of the MMR/autism story. When looking more specifically at the coverage of single vaccines and not looking just at whether they are mentioned, 55% of stories state that single jabs *should* be offered and parents *should* have a choice. The case against single jabs, and hence of limiting parental choice, was difficult to make in a limited amount of time. The frame constructed and news values emphasised placed the burden of proof on the side of those defending the MMR vaccine.[6] The case against single vaccinations is three-fold: all the empirical data suggests that MMR is safe, the time lapse between three separate injections (Wakefield recommended a year) increases the likelihood of infant infection, and thirdly, unlike MMR, there is no research on why three separate vaccines are safer (British Medical Association 2003).

The instinct of journalists to follow the lead set by other media outlets, 'pack journalism', means only one media outlet need deem a story to have news values and then others will follow. The *Daily Mail* has been a powerful influence on the Labour government on many issues since New Labour won its first election in 1997 as it was in the MMR/autism story. One journalist, when asked why the MMR vaccine was such a big story, answered:

I think a lot of it is the *Daily Mail* who are very anti-it. If you look at all the research, the original research is based on 12 children and hasn't been repeated all over the world. And nowhere else but this country does anybody link it with Crohn's disease or autism. It's only in this country.

(Popular health editor)

When BBC journalist Roger Harrabin interviewed journalists about health and risk stories several 'pointed to the *Daily Mail* as a powerful source of "news" for other newspapers and for broadcast news. Its campaign against the MMR vaccine was cited as an irresistible story that had to be pursued as "news"' (Harrabin et al. 2003: 32). The editor of the BBC 10 o'clock news, Mark Popescu, claimed the controversy over MMR would continue across the media as long as the *Daily Mail* kept running with the story (ibid.). When one journalist argued with his colleagues about following the agenda set by other media outlets, he claimed the *Daily Mail* was a 'crucial factor' in keeping the story alive.

The pack instinct in journalism is now frightening. There is no way you could say, once the ball starts rolling, there is no way you can say 'This story is not worth doing, let's not do it'...If the *Mail* splashes 'New doubts about MMR vaccine' I'll end up doing the story even if it's utter crap—I'll end up doing it.

(Television health and science editor)

In response, the *Daily Mail* claims it is simply reporting a scientific controversy, and one of their journalists stated the *Mail* was merely concerned with:

...strong stories that would have a resonance with (our) readers...Some of these might appear to be scare stories – but if they have a certain basis in science, they make news. Our readers are adults and they can decide for themselves how scared they ought to be. Of course in empirical terms we do go over the top from time to time – and there might be all sorts of reasons for that...but if people didn't like the paper's coverage they wouldn't buy it.

(in Harrabin et al. 2003: 54)

Whilst another *Daily Mail* journalist offered a different motivation:

Health scares are part of the price you pay for an open democratic society in which a free press plays a crucial part.

(ibid.)

Not all journalists agreed the *Daily Mail* held such power over other media outlets; one argued it only covered MMR 'when something new happens' (Broadsheet health editor).

The media analysis reflects the findings from the journalists' interviews that pack journalism was influential in the MMR/autism story—there are frequent examples of cross-referencing between the media. The *Today* programme regularly used newspapers as a hook for their own stories. On 6 February 2002 they begin a story about the MMR vaccine with an interview with Trevor Kavanagh, political editor of *The Sun*. They discuss his claim in the paper that Leo Blair had received single vaccines and later used this to challenge the junior health minister at the time, Yvette Cooper.

> Where did Trevor Kavanagh get this from? He's a very respectable as you know, very respected, I don't know whether he's respectable but he's certainly respected political editor and he doesn't get stories wrong by and large.
>
> (John Humphries, *Today* BBC radio 6 February 2002)

The *Today* programme often uses newspapers as a source of information:

> I don't know if you've seen the papers yet this morning but the *Mail* and the *Independent* are leading with the story, other papers have got it as well, that Tony Blair's son Leo has had the jab now. He was given it last week. They're reporting that now they haven't given a source for that but um, but reporting it quite authoritatively as it were.
>
> (John Humphries, *Today* BBC radio 2 February 2002)

At the same time, the *Today* programme acts as an agenda-setter for the rest of the media. For example, when Dr. Paul Shattock appeared on the *Today* programme to publicise research (not yet peer-reviewed) on 27 June 2002, a number of media outlets (*Daily Mail, The Guardian, The Sun, Mail on Sunday, Daily Telegraph, Sunday Times*) picked up the story the next day. Some journalists do not even bother to contact the source and use the *Today* programme for direct quotes.

> Peter Dukes, of the Medical Research Council, yesterday told BBC Radio 4's *Today* programme that Mr Shattock should "publish his research and come forward to the MRC with positive proposals".
>
> (*The Guardian* 28 June 2002)

Referring to stories appearing elsewhere in the media allowed the media to keep the story on the news agenda without doing research themselves. Both pack journalism and editorial agendas gave the MMR/autism story continuing news value.

Framing Health and Science as Political, Not Scientific

Whilst the MMR/autism story is inherently scientific, scientific angles did not dominate. Instead, the media analysis showed that the MMR story was, above all, a political story, a political controversy. Wakefield's research released in 2002 (Uhlmann et al. 2002) was only used as a hook in a little over 10% of the stories; instead, political events, vaccination levels dropping and measles outbreaks were more likely to attract coverage. More than three-quarters of all stories reported the MMR/autism story with little reference to science or research and instead concentrated on what journalists considered more newsworthy: politics, the call for choice in vaccinations and the risks and dangers of the measles outbreaks (see Table 3.1). Content analysis of the most popular science stories found that the best way to engage the public is to make it less a science story and avoid lengthy scientific explanations (Boyce et al. 2007, Hargreaves and Ferguson 2000: 52).

Table 3.1 Story themes and leads (N=285)

Story type	Theme	Lead
Political	26%	26%
Call for choice/single vaccines	20%	15%
Outbreaks/vaccination dropping	13%	17%
New research pro-Wakefield	9%	10%
Parental reaction	11%	0%
Personal experience	0%	6%
Autism	3%	6%
Other	6%	5%
New research anti-Wakefield	4%	3%
Call to vaccinate	4%	0%
Dangers of disease	0%	4%
Dangers of vaccine	0%	3%
Background/history	4%	2%
Legal cases	0%	2%

Stories that had the main theme as scientific, primarily covering research, accounted for only 13% of the stories. The difference between the level of pro- and anti-MMR research is another example of how the anti-MMR research was made more p7rominent. Table 3.1 shows pro-Wakefield research was the theme and lead in many more stories than research challenging his claims.

In line with the dominant story theme, political leads were the most common lead. Half of all stories led with one of three stories: a political angle, the measles outbreaks or the drop in vaccination levels. Again, science issues do not typically appear in the lead and were not used to try to attract the public to the story.

Whilst new research by Andrew Wakefield published in February 2002 led to a small flourish of articles, the reason behind the surge of coverage at the beginning of 2002 was a political story; the media's obsession with the vaccination status of Leo Blair, the Prime Minister's youngest son. This aspect provided political news values and made the MMR/autism story not about science, but about trusting the Prime Minister and trusting politicians. Leo Blair was discussed in 32% of the stories but the differences between the media reveal the differing news values of each outlet. For example, the BBC radio *Today* programme steered clear of the Leo Blair story; it appears in only 13% of all stories compared to 36% on the two television bulletins, 35% broadsheets and 31% in tabloids. The following *Sun* article written by its *political* (not health) editor and headlined MUMS 'ARE WINNING MMR WAR' demonstrates how politics came to dominate the MMR/autism story. The article's tone and angle are set in the first two sentences:

> Here we can see the patronising attitude of the MMR PR – just take it, it's safe, denying the worries of parents. MUMS have pushed Tony Blair on to the defensive over MMR by shunning the vaccine in record numbers.

Also typical in this article are the sources selected: 1 scientist, 1 government department representative, 2 politicians and 2 parents – clearly this was less about science than politics. As the article continues, a public health doctor appeals to expert scientific opinion and this is followed by the Health Minister, whose views are then criticised by an opposition *politician:*

> ...Gill Sanders, director of public health for Gateshead and South Tyneside, said: "The message is that MMR is safe, it is backed by health practitioners, but it is not being accepted by some parents. Because of the success of immunisation, nobody has seen the suffering that measles causes. We need to get over a positive message to parents that MMR is safe and the risk of measles could be avoided. Parents don't need to worry and should take up the MMR vaccine for their children. If you are looking for the best quality and

cost-effective treatment then it is MMR." Health Secretary Alan Milburn also battled to reassure parents, saying: "I know there are real concerns but the vaccine is the safest way of protecting children against what can be potentially life-threatening conditions. "If I thought there was a safer alternative to MMR I would sanction it." The Department of Health also insisted the recent outbreaks were "not unusual" and added: "There are about 100 measles outbreaks each year." Shadow Health Secretary Dr Liam Fox said the Government's policy was "a public health disaster." He added: "As ever, the real victims are likely to be innocent children rather than inept ministers."...

The article ends in classic tabloid style, with the appearance of frustrated readers, who are described as trying to make sense of a world where politicians and expert-sources like scientists are constantly lying to them and where the newspaper is the hero:

> The combined injection costs £60 compared to £200 for individual shots. The Sun was flooded with messages yesterday backing our call for free single jabs. Reader Nigel Furniss, who has a 13-month-old daughter, asked: "Does Tony Blair know how much damage he's doing by failing to say whether his child has had the MMR jab?" Mum Helen Moorey, from Gloucestershire, said: "Both my older children had problems after having their MMR jabs. My youngest daughter is ten months old. I don't want her to have MMR but I am now terrified she will catch measles after this outbreak."
>
> (*The Sun* 6 February 2002)

Whilst this is only one article, it is typical in many ways of how the MMR story was covered; political accusations were met with defensive scientific statements and scientific assurances were challenged by political arguments.

All sources interviewed agreed Tony Blair's refusal to state Leo's vaccination status had a significant impact on how the story was reported and the amount of coverage the MMR/autism story received. Those sources who were representatives of medical organisations agreed the Prime Minster had a right to patient confidentiality.

> We did work out quite a strong line on (Leo) and it was about patient confidentiality. And it was that they had the right to privacy that child, like anybody, has the right to privacy...I'm sure the child has had it, that's the irony. But it's a red herring and it sort of fuels paranoia.
>
> (Royal College)

When the Medical Research Council (MRC) published a substantial review of the causes and epidemiology of autism in December 2001 they stated the 'big media furore' that resulted from the report was due to the fact Leo Blair was then approaching the MMR vaccination age[7], which journalists used as a hook when covering the report's findings.

The extent to which this story was politicised is exemplified in the following example, where a mother in one of the focus groups imagines an image that does not appear once in the sample:

> The thing that struck me was, you had the argument for it and the argument against it but it was never really put together in a sort of logical way for you to think right, ok…You'd read the newspaper and you'd get the against side but you'd never really see anything, bar some stuffed shirt outside Downing Street, saying 'oh it's really good' and you kinda don't believe those people anyway.
>
> (V5[8])

Whilst this parent claims to be influenced by the image that never happens in the sample (and unlikely to happen as the DoH knows from its own research that these images are likely to increase distrust, as the quote indicates), suggesting the extent to which the pro-MMR side was linked to the government rather than to science. This dichotomy fits the framework that the MMR vaccine has been politicised and that it is politicians and bureaucrats doling out medical advice and not scientists.

The role of columnists is to possess strong opinions and prompt political debate. Both journalists and columnists used their personal experience when covering the MMR/autism story and this further encouraged the political frame. Columnists like Suzanne Moore at the *Mail on Sunday* repeatedly returned to what she labelled as an 'agonising' decision about whether or not to vaccinate their child:

> It is sad, I know, but for some time now I have been waiting for a sign from God or at least Tony Blair about what to do. I was set to give my daughter the MMR jab—my other kids have had it—when she contracted meningitis. She recovered, but after such a trauma I am reluctant to do anything that might endanger her health. Like so many other parents, I am waiting, I suppose, for some final reassurance that this thing really is safe.
>
> (*Mail on Sunday* 30 June 2002)

Columnists typically included MMR in a list of blunders by the Prime Minister and only rarely addressed wider issues concerning science. The following Alice Thomson column is typical as to how the MMR jab appeared in lists of mistakes made by the government.

> Mr Blair pretends to take "personal charge", but always finds scapegoats. Foot and mouth: let's sack Nick Brown. Welfare reform: there goes Harriet

Harman and Frank Field. Transport: Stephen Byers obviously isn't up to it. MMR: it's over-protective parents' fault.

(*Daily Telegraph* 15 February 2002)

Few columnists reflected the frustration of parents and instead focused on the political controversy. In a rare example of media accounts reflecting the confusion of parents, guest columnist Carey Scott in the *Sunday Times* comments:

> We have come to a strange pass when parents are made to feel they have a cavalier attitude to their children's health because they follow government advice on vaccinating their children. No, I hadn't gone on the internet and surfed my way across every single website on MMR. I don't have a science degree either, so I hadn't read every study ever published in a medical journal. I had worked out that I trusted my GP and my health visitor, and I asked them what they thought, read reports on the issue and then weighed up the facts. And like most parents in Britain, my husband and I decided that our child, Matilda, should be vaccinated on schedule at 13 months. The fact that, since 84.2% of British children are vaccinated with MMR, we are part of a vast majority seems to have been forgotten amid the hysteria of recent days.

(*Sunday Times* 10 February 2002)

Over half of all columns and 21% of all stories mention the MMR vaccine only once, suggesting that columnists were using the MMR/autism story to make wider political points (see Table 3.2).

Table 3.2 Columnists' (daily/weekly) views on the MMR vaccine

Pro-MMR	Anti-MMR
Paul Routledge *The Mirror*	Pippa Sibley *The Mirror*
Suzanne Moore *Mail on Sunday*	Peter Hitchens *Mail on Sunday*
	Lauren Booth *Mail on Sunday*
	Quentin Letts *Daily Mail*
	Lynda Lee Potter *Daily Mail*
	Colette Douglas-Home *Daily Mail*
	Robert Harris *Daily Telegraph*
	Catherine Bennett (soft) *The Guardian*

Columnists were more likely to be anti-MMR, with five columnists from the *Daily Mail* and *Mail on Sunday* writing against the MMR vaccine. These non-news stories were important in keeping the MMR/autism story in the news pages and not the science sections.

Risk, Trust and Blame

Science and health stories that can tap into society's obsession with trust and risk are more attractive to journalists. Instead of reporting these stories simply within a health or science frame, journalists use trust and risk to attract audiences and make a story newsworthy. That we are now living in a 'risk society' is a common theme in contemporary society and the media's increasing attention to health stories can be viewed as evidence of our obsession with risk. Ulrich Beck's (1992) Risk Society thesis has become the most influential theory assessing risk and modernity. For Beck, wealth no longer defines society; instead anxiety is the distinguishing feature of the modern risk society. Beck's Risk Society thesis has its strengths in providing an alternateve to post-modernism however, it has its shortcomings. The thesis rarely refers to the media; where it does, it has been criticised for a simplistic understanding and analysis (see, for instance, Mythen 2004, Cottle 1998). Beck's theories are useful in applying a wider, theoretical framework and understanding why risk debates dominate Western societies. For more valuable research relevant to media studies, Jenny Kitzinger provides a media-centric analysis of *how* and *why* risks are covered (or not) in the media, and considers issues related to media content, production issues and audience theories. She criticises established risk society theories for failing to 'provide a thorough analysis of processes of media production or to present empirical evidence of how media coverage develops' (1999a: 67).

Kitzinger's review of risk research (1999a) analysed not only whether risk is amplified or attenuated, but also wider issues concerning the way risk is reported. The MMR/autism story corresponds well to the factors highlighted by Kitzinger in her review and provides explanation as to why the MMR/autism story received substantial media coverage.

For example, in examining the *nature* of risks, Kitzinger concludes positive findings of risk are more likely to receive coverage. In the MMR/autism story Wakefield's claims linking the MMR vaccine to autism received more coverage, and more *prominent* coverage, than research finding no link. She also finds scientific controversy is more attractive than uncertainty; in the MMR/autism story the controversial aspects of Wakefield's accusations were emphasised, not the uncertainty of the MMR/autism link.

The strength of Kitzinger's research is her acknowledgment of the role of production factors and media dynamics in media coverage of risks. As Beck's risk society thesis is not grounded in practical examples like Kitzinger's work, he is unable to conclude, for instance, that strong visual images increase the chance of a risk being reported, as Kitzinger (1999a) discovered. This factor affected how the MMR/autism story was reported: images of children being vaccinated at single vaccine clinics were frequently used as a backdrop in television news. The status quo and therefore less controversial image of children being vaccinated by the MMR vaccine, was not used once by television in the sample analysed.

The ability to blame someone also gives a story more news values, and this increases the possibility of a risk being reported. In this story Wakefield, opposition politicians and campaigning news outlets all blamed the government for not offering single vaccines.

The 'carrying capacity' of different media formats influences the news values in risk stories. Women's pages, health sections and parent sections in newspapers all carried stories about the MMR vaccine, even when the story was not at the top of the news agenda. The carrying capacity of newspapers had more of an influence in the level of coverage of the MMR/autism story than the actual scientific developments or research. Fifty percent of the newspaper articles appeared after page 10 and one-quarter of all articles were not news stories but were editorials, features, columns or letters to agony aunts—this was a story that could easily act as a filler.

Kitzinger's review identifies how risk stories shift and change because of production factors.[9] For example, reporting of a risk will shift over time due to story fatigue, as journalists and audiences tire of the warnings. Table 1.1 in Chapter 1 (page 6) shows the decline in MMR/autism stories since 1998 as Wakefield remains one of very few scientists making the MMR/autism link.

Media dynamics is the most important factor to understand why the MMR/autism story was covered and explains the type of coverage it received. In Kitzinger's review she argues the reporting of a risk is influenced by journalists' 'mental maps' and how they frame a story. As established, the impact of BSE on the MMR/autism story was immense and this is one of the key media dynamics influencing how the story was reported and which news values journalists used most frequently. In interviews journalists stated they viewed this as another government scientific cover-up and was similar to the BSE/CJD crisis. Kitzinger also identifies that particular attention is given to a risk because of journalists' personal identification with the threat. Many journalists, particularly columnists, openly identified as parents making the decision over whether to use the MMR vaccine. Media interest feeding off itself, or pack journalism, is another media dynamic Kitzinger identifies and, as established earlier in this chapter, the *Daily Mail* exerted a strong influence in the MMR/autism story.

When looking more specifically at how risks are covered it is clear journalists chose to emphasise the risk from the vaccine over the risks from the three diseases the vaccine offers protection from (see Figure 3.1). Parents were therefore more likely to read or hear about the risks from the vaccine rather than the risks from one of the diseases.

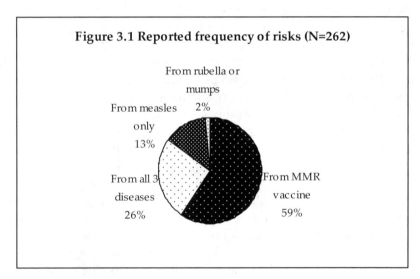

Figure 3.1 Reported frequency of risks (N=262)

One of the ways in which journalists made the risk from the vaccine appear more real was to emphasise and possibly exaggerate the emotional state of parents.

> Yet panic has gripped much of the nation. Perfectly sensible parents are terrified that they are threatening the health of their infants if they give them the triple jab.
>
> (*The Mirror* 7 February 2002)

Threats and risks to children have added news value. Risk stories about children contain more news values because of the potential of 'innocent' victims. A number of journalists agreed the story attracted attention because it was about children's health.

> When you think that you're injecting a child with something that's going to cause them damage it becomes very worrying for parents. There's nothing more worried than a parent.
>
> (General news correspondent)

> It's a good story because most people out there who are reading it are parents or grandparents.
>
> (Royal College)

Headlines are significant in any study of newspapers, as they are usually read first, are often the only part of the article consumed and have a high recall rate (van Dijk 1991: 50-51). Headlines emphasised the fear and controversy of the MMR vaccine. The aim of the sub-editor, who usually writes the headlines, is to summarise and attract the reader to stories; they therefore select what they think is the most newsworthy aspect in the article (Bell 1991: 189). 'Fear' was the most common verb in headlines, appearing in 21 headlines. Verbs were more likely to emphasise the claimed 'dangers' of the MMR vaccine rather than supporting its safety (see Figure 3.2).

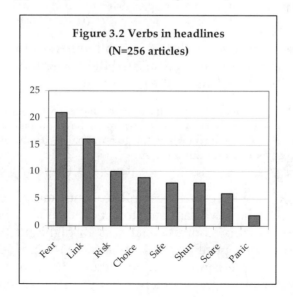

Figure 3.2 Verbs in headlines (N=256 articles)

Verbs like 'fear' and 'risk' were more often attached to the MMR vaccine and not to measles, mumps or rubella, with headlines such as:

Fear of MMR jab sparks measles outbreak: Research raises new MMR questions

(*The Guardian* 6 February 2002)

RISK OF MISSING TRIPLE INJECTION

(*The Sun* 6 February 2002)

MMR SCARE IN U.S.; DOCTOR CLAIMS NEW RESEARCH ADDS TO AUTISM LINK THEORY

(*The Mirror* 9 August 2002)

On the whole, journalists were interested in issues concerning trust because of the commanding frame provided by the BSE crisis. The newsworthiness of the story centred around the distrust of the government and the medical establishment and *as a result of this distrust*, risk issues arose. As the editor of the BBC News at 10, Mark Popescu, admits, distrust of the government made the story newsworthy, not the scientific risks:

…strictly on the level of risk, we probably over-reported MMR but I am not just governed by that cold calculation. I am also governed by whether there is a public debate going on, whether the Government is involved, whether the Chief Medical Officer is involved and whether things are being said by all of those people, which I have a responsibility to report as well.

(in Harrabin et al. 2003: 31)

When discussing risk, journalists frequently referred to the declining trust in government advice. They argued the MMR/autism story highlighted society's lack of trust in the government.

It's a bigger issue… about trust with the government…A lot of my criticism has been to do with the way the government have mishandled the issue…MMR is but one issue on which the government seems unable to listen to people in any kind of reassuring (way).

(Newspaper columnist)

Leo Blair's vaccination record was an excellent example of how trust was used to give the MMR/autism story news values. The way journalists made this story controversial was to highlight the inconsistency in Tony Blair's position. Blair maintained this was a personal matter, but for people confused about who to trust, this was an important indicator of the government's faith in its own position. Was the government's support for MMR deeply felt or merely tactical and strategic? The media chose to frame Leo Blair as a reasonable test of the government's confidence in its own position. *The Daily Mail* emphasises this in the following article:

> Parental concern over MMR measles, mumps and rubella has grown since Tony Blair refused to say whether or not his son Leo had had the triple jab. His silence fuelled speculation that Leo had received single jabs or had not been vaccinated at all.
>
> (*Daily Mail* 1 July 2002)

The Prime Minister's refusal to state his son Leo's vaccination status was viewed by sources as exemplifying how trust had become a problem for the government and scientists. GP Mike Fitzpatrick labels Blair's 'equivocal response (as) probably the most significant public relations setback for MMR since Dr. Wakefield's initial allegations' (2004: 28). Journalists agreed that the Leo Blair episode resonated with their audience, who could relate to the Blair's parental predicament.

> I think it (the story) would've died if Blair had said that Leo had been vaccinated...I heard lots of people say to me, if the case for MMR is so compelling and he's had his own child vaccinated, why doesn't he tell us... I think the fact that he wouldn't say so led to a lot of nudging and winks in pubs and clubs and on the tube and on the bus and all the rest of it and people saying 'Oh there must be something funny here otherwise why doesn't he say?'...People just say, 'Well why didn't the Prime Minister say?'
>
> (Science editor)

The campaigning newspapers took every opportunity to blame the government, not science, for the declining MMR uptake. For example, the *Mail* and *Sun* framed parents as unconvinced of the safety of the MMR vaccine because of *government ministers'* pronouncements, not advice from their health practitioners.

> A third of parents in the area have refused the vaccine for their children over fears it is linked to autism and bowel disease, in spite of repeated assurances from Ministers over its safety.
>
> (*Daily Mail* 23 February 2002)

> MMR has been linked to bowel disease and autism, though the Government has repeatedly insisted the jab is safe.
>
> (*The Sun* 29 March 2002)

The news values in this story—controversy, the politics of science, editorial agendas and risk and trust—are examples of news values specific to health and science stories. These categories attempt to explain why some health and science stories are covered by journalists whilst other research languishes in peer-reviewed journals. The news values in the MMR/autism story tended to emphasise the arguments of the anti-MMR side and put the pro-MMR side on the defensive. The news values in this story provide the first indication as to how the anti-MMR side was made more prominent in media coverage. The following chapter provides further evidence of the anti-MMR argument being more prominent and analyses the effect balance had on the MMR/autism story.

CHAPTER FOUR

Balance in Health and Science Stories

Notions of balance continue to dominate contemporary journalism. It is still taught as best practice in journalism schools and is commonly regarded by journalists as a signifier that a story is fair. Balance is regarded as *proof* that journalists and journalism are not biased, demonstrating that a journalist is not under the influence of a source or purporting a certain angle. Balanced stories, however, do not always result in 'objective' reporting. This is a particularly important point in science, health and risk stories when new research challenges the status quo or when the bulk of scientific evidence is on one side (e.g., climate change). Because so-called 'balanced' stories can still contain bias therefore, useful research into the role balance plays is not simply about identifying which sides of a debate are reported and needs to be more comprehensive. In the MMR/autism story the dependence on balance significantly influenced how the story was reported and framed and, crucially, how it was received by the audience.[1]

In the UK newspaper market, balance has a particular definition, for each newspaper has a distinct editorial leaning—either to the left (*The Guardian, Independent, Mirror*) or the right (*Daily Telegraph, The Times, The Sun, Daily Mail, Daily Express*). Within these political leanings, these papers aim to balanced reporting but often do so by consistently putting one side on the defensive (e.g., the *Daily Mail* will be more lenient on the Conservative Party than the Labour Party or the *Express*'s anti-refugee/immigrant stance). Television and radio news in the UK reflects that found in countries like the USA and Canada and aims to be balanced without overt political leanings. The publicly funded BBC is passionate about 'balance' and it is written into their Code of Practice for journalists to follow. Although these media outlets claim to have a formal commitment to balance, nonetheless certain views do predominate. For example, the benefits of capitalism and globalisation dictate coverage of labour and financial stories (see, for example, Kumar 2007, Herman and Chomsky 1988, Glasgow Media Group 1976, 1980, 1982).

The Relationship Between Objectivity and Balance

Defining the relationship between objectivity and balance requires clear definitions. Balance is the absence of bias in a story but how 'bias' is defined is less clear (Starkey 2006). Journalists claim an absence of bias means they have reported objectively. Tuchman's influential work in the 1970s showed journalists follow the 'strategic ritual of objectivity' to defend themselves against accusations of bias. Because objectivity is routine and thus hegemonic, Tuchman argues journalists write balanced stories and thus believe they are unbiased. Other researchers argue journalists use objectivity as a guide because 'true' objectivity is not possible and therefore a balanced story is the closest one can get to 'true' objectivity (Manning 2001).

The belief that including 'both' sides of a story automatically leads to a bias-free or balanced story is problematic. The convention of balanced reporting can lead to biased stories when covering stories where not all sides are equal or when there are more than two sides to a story, as is often the case. Balanced stories can create the appearance of a conflict when there is not two equal amounts of evidence. 'Seeking balance works perfectly well in those situations where the issue is one-dimensional' (Merritt 1995: 375), but most stories are much more complex than this. The quest for objective stories controls journalists' behaviour by influencing source selection and how stories are framed. In Croteau and Hoynes' study of the ABC news magazine *Nightline* they argue the adherence to balance:

> ...is often more illusory than real...If balance is having two people, usually elites or experts, disagreeing over fine points rather than a range of guests arguing fundamental questions, then *Nightline* presents a balanced guest list. In reality, *Nightline*'s observance of the balance norm obscures the fact that there are stark imbalances.
>
> (1994: 100)

When journalists reduce a story to only two perspectives this results in complex issues being reduced to simple conflicts between two opposing parties (see, for example, Mormont and Dasnoy 1995: 61, Dunwoody 1999, Singer and Endreny 1993: 15, Stocking 1999).

Related to this is another reason why balance is useful to journalists. Journalists without the expertise or time to research complex issues frame a story as an argument between two sides and can then claim it is fair and objective, even if they are unsure of the details. This reliance on balance and presenting each story as only possessing two sides can lead to 'a good deal of autopilot reporting and lazy thinking' where journalists become more interested in 'presenting' stories and not reporting them (Joan Didion in Cunningham 2003: 28). Balanced stories become didactic (Bennett et al. 1985: 51) as stories are debated between two opinions, excluding those who speak outside the two defined sides. For instance, in media coverage about stem cell research, Williams et al. argue that 'in spite, or even *because*, of the apparently 'balanced' nature of media coverage it systematically marginalises women's perspectives, disregards more fundamental challenges to science, and curtails discussion of broader social and political issues' (2003: 794 emphasis in original, see also Cunningham 2003: 26). Thus, even when journalists balance a story, it can still contain bias, by, for example, consistently presenting one side first or by framing one side as responding to another's accusations—both of which are evident in the MMR/autism story.

The Challenge of Balance in Science/Health Stories

When reporting science and health stories there are additional complexities concerning balance. One of the main criticisms made of science and medicine reporting is journalists' 'commitment to balance' (Kitzinger 1999a) when scientific evidence is so rarely equally balanced. This is particularly taxing for journalists when covering the views of so-called 'maverick' scientists. Journalists' commitment to balance leads to equal weight being given to majority and fringe scientists and to scientists and non-scientists (e.g., Stocking 1999 and Dearing 1994). The lone voice of one source can receive equal coverage to the rest of the scientific community with:

'(t)he net result of these processes may be a spurious image of equally valid opposing positions…if there is no 'weighting' by either the relative frequency with which (opinions) are held or the quality of evidence on which (opinions) are based, may convey an inaccurate, even biased, picture of knowledge in a field'. (Singer and Endreny 1993: 15)

Equating and reporting the claims of a small minority of scientists with the scientific community does not result in a 'balanced' story, free of bias; instead the evidence should be weighed so that the *evidence* is not balanced. A prominent theme in research from health professionals in the MMR/autism story is the undue weight given to Andrew Wakefield's research, or as Ramsay et al. state:

> 'the extent of media interest in the potential side effects of MMR has been disproportionate to the weight of negative evidence...sufficient weight has not been given to the positive evidence that allows redress of the balance in favour of MMR'. (2002: 915)

Thus, the convention of balancing advantages 'maverick' scientists. Journalists' commitment to balance is 'ill-suited to communicating scientific theories that have not received widespread support among scientists to general audiences' (Dearing 1994: 343). Journalists' concepts of balance are less influenced by the number of studies published and are instead influenced more by professional practices, like balancing a story by using an equal number of sources.

In coverage of science and health stories, *over-balancing* is often a problem when new evidence challenges the status quo or when maverick scientists use the media to secure coverage. Over-balancing occurs when stories are equally balanced even though the research is not. When two opposing points of view are reported as equally plausible yet one has 'the preponderance of reason and evidence on its side' we have what has been termed a *charade of objectivity* (Lichtenberg 1996: 240). *Under-balancing,* when journalists fail to report or acknowledge parts of the debate and only report one side of a story, can also have implications on how stories are reported. Because science, health and risk stories are often very complicated, journalists frequently use only the source from the press releases and depend on science processes such as peer review to help determine a story's validity (Stocking 1999). But, if stories which are balanced or over-balanced or under-balanced can all lead to biased reporting—what approach should journalists take? Levi offers advice for some of these stories when he suggests '(journalists) are supposed to weigh the information, not to balance it' (2001: 34). Including an evaluation of the weight of scientific research does offer a partial solution but also to be addressed is the practice of weighting sources. In the MMR/autism story the practice of balancing and over-balancing evidence and sources had powerful influences on how the story was reported and received.

Balancing *Evidence* in the MMR/Autism Story

The initial analysis of balance placed each story in one of three categories:

- Balanced (including pro- and anti-MMR information);
- Pro-MMR only;
- Anti-MMR only.[2]

Half of all stories in the corpus were balanced including both anti- and pro-MMR sides, one-third contained only the anti-MMR argument and one-fifth the pro-MMR argument (see Figure 4.1).

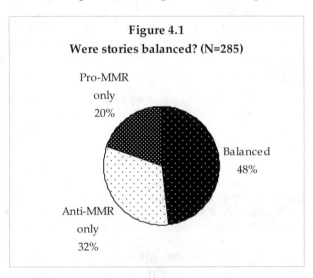

Figure 4.1
Were stories balanced? (N=285)

Pro-MMR only 20%

Balanced 48%

Anti-MMR only 32%

That half of all stories were balanced does not provide explanation as to how these balanced stories weighed more heavily on the anti-MMR side. Of the balanced stories the anti-MMR side was made more prominent in a number of ways. Although many stories were 'balanced' and included both sides of the argument, often the pro-MMR side was physically given less space than the anti-MMR sources. In a story appearing on the front page and page 4, the *Daily Mail* writes of the increase in measles cases and the dangers of the disease. The first quote is given to a pressure group representative (chief executive of the Patients' Association) who claims that 'People have lost confidence in the vaccination and there are so many new pieces of evidence coming forward'. The article then quotes two doctors calling for a public inquiry into the MMR vaccine, a reference to research which suggests 'one in every 1,500 injections with the combined jab could trigger autism' but provides no further detail. Jackie Fletcher from JABS then states 'parents are concerned and we have more than 2,000 families with children we say have been damaged by MMR. More studies are questioning the safety of MMR, yet the Government insists it is safe'—the first presence of the pro-MMR argument, but appearing after a statement of its danger. For the next 450 words the article discusses the difficulties of securing single vaccines and the article then finishes with these last three paragraphs:

> Concern over MMR and autism first emerged in 1998, when British researcher Dr Andrew Wakefield diagnosed a bowel disease in autistic children which has been linked to MMR. U.S. studies have since appeared to back up his findings. Last week Dr Arthur Krigsman, a paediatric gastroenterologist from New York University, told a Congressional committee on autism that he had found an identical pattern of inflammatory bowel disease in 90 per cent of his young autistic patients.

> At the same time, Paul Shattock, director of Sunderland's University's Autism Research Unit, revealed that he had found abnormalities in urine samples from autistic children whose parents believe they were affected by MMR. He said his results suggested that the vaccine is responsible for ten per cent of autism, a rate of one case per 1,500 jabs.

> The Department of Health, however, insists that MMR is the safest way to protect children and there is no firm evidence of links to autism or bowel disease. A spokesman said it was keeping new evidence under review.
> ('MEASLES SOAR AS PARENTS SAY NO TO MMR' *Daily Mail* 1 July 2002)

Those defending the vaccine are given minimal space and, in this 1,000+ word article, are given the final sentence and 28 words to state the vaccine is safe. The article might be balanced, but there is explicit emphasis on the alleged dangers of the MMR vaccine.

In another example, the following short article includes both the pro- and anti-arguments; however, it is the MMR vaccine which is on the defensive. Wakefield's claim of a link between the MMR vaccine and autism is exaggerated; he refers to research not yet published as proof and the only direct quote is given to Wakefield, who makes a plea for a nebulous 'new attitude' whilst the journalist chose not to allow the DoH a rebuttal.

> THE doctor who first raised concerns about MMR has been asked by the Health Department to turn his research over for independent analysis. Dr Andrew Wakefield's work suggests a connection between the jab and autism

and bowel disease. He claims studies this year will show a link. His research contradicts the department's view that MMR is safe. Dr Wakefield said: "Let's hope this is the start of a new attitude to this serious dilemma."

(The Sun 18 February 2002)

Consistently, these supposedly balanced stories place the burden of proof on those *defending* the MMR vaccine, such as the following from *ITV* news:

John Draper (ITV): In tonight's poll most respondents think that Tony Blair should go public. 80% also want alternatives to MMR. This Liverpool clinic does just that—offering single jabs for each disease to worried parents.

Parent: You should be able to have your children vaccinated singly at your own doctors. I object strongly to being told what and when to inject into my children.

Dr Pat Troop, Deputy Chief Medical Officer: We have no concerns about our current vaccine. I think it will send a very strong signal that parents will say, hang on we think that maybe there is a problem around this vaccine— why else would you offer us a single vaccine—and confidence would go.

(ITV news 4 February 2002)

What is missing from much of the coverage is any sense of the *weight* of scientific evidence, which is firmly stacked on the side of the safety of the MMR vaccine.

When examining balance, it is not simply a matter of counting which side appeared more often, but balance is also influenced by how journalists used scientific evidence. Journalists selected almost equal numbers of scientists for and against the MMR vaccine, suggesting that scientists were evenly split on this issue, when in reality, the vast majority of scientists and health professionals supported the MMR vaccine (see Figure 4.2). Journalists used parents to *question* the vaccine's safety but very rarely used them to *support* the vaccine.

Anti-MMR discourse still prevailed in stories even when all sources were pro-MMR with the statements between sources providing the anti-MMR discourse. For example, in a front page article the *Daily Mail* uses the Health Secretary to defend the vaccine but the text emphasises the dangers of the vaccine, even though the scientific evidence and sources were 'balanced'.

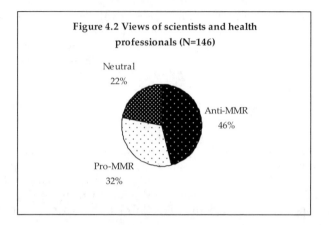

Figure 4.2 Views of scientists and health professionals (N=146)

Neutral 22%

Anti-MMR 46%

Pro-MMR 32%

The front-page article begins with an accusation against the triple jab:

'NEW ALERT ON MMR JAB'

NEW research fuelled controversy over the MMR jab yesterday as fears grew of a large-scale measles outbreak. *Scientists have for the first time established a possible link between the measles virus, autism and a related bowel disorder.* The findings were revealed as clusters of measles, which can be fatal, emerged in London and the North-East.

Public health experts warned that record numbers of parents are shunning the combined measles, mumps and rubella jab. The proportion of children being vaccinated is well below the critical threshold at which epidemics become a serious risk.

The latest research shows that the measles virus is present in the guts of autistic children who suffer a rare form of bowel disease. The disorder was first identified by Dr Andrew Wakefield, the expert who voiced fears about a link between MMR and autism in 1998. *Some experts believe measles may act as a 'trigger' to the children's immune systems and cause the inflammatory bowel disease.* The research, to be published in the respected Molecular Pathology journal of the British Medical Association, dealt a further blow to the Government's campaign to persuade parents MMR is safe.

Health Secretary Alan Milburn insisted: 'The vaccine is the safest way of protecting children against what can be life-threatening conditions. If I thought there was a safer alternative I would sanction it.' But there were renewed calls for the Government to fund independent studies into the safety of MMR and to make single vaccines available on the NHS.

(emphasis added *Daily Mail* 6 February 2002)

Note that the three sentences in italics do not state the MMR vaccine is to blame, but the measles virus. Whether the virus is naturally occurring or the result of the MMR vaccine is not established in the research; however, the blame in the headline and first sentence is on the MMR vaccine.

Under-balancing frequently appeared in campaigning newspapers such as the *Daily Mail* and *The Sun*, which consistently emphasised anti-MMR frames. For example, a *Daily Mail* story was five times more likely to only use the anti-MMR argument rather than include only the pro-MMR 'side' (see Table 4.1). In often short articles, parents' claims against the MMR vaccine went uncontested; any notions of objectivity were clearly not a concern, as the following example suggests:

> Mother-of-three Pouli Otton yesterday called for single jabs on the NHS. Her daughters Natasha four, and Eleanor two, attend White House School and have had single jabs, while baby Alfred, eight months, stays at home and has not been immunised yet. She said: "The whole thing makes me really cross. I don't know how people can refute the link the evidence suggests between MMR and autism."
>
> (*Daily Mail* 14 February 2002)

In the *Daily Mail* the safety of the MMR vaccine was rarely stated; this occurred in only 7% of stories, whereas in the *Mail on Sunday* every article either overtly doubted the safety of the triple jab or balanced the arguments for and against the vaccine. When these outlets decided to back Wakefield's theories and challenge the government's stance, they did so consistently. Table 4.1 shows just how political this science story had become, with the anti-Labour papers so clearly anti-MMR. Table 4.1 also reveals the BBC's commitment to balanced reportage. The two outlets most likely to have balanced stories are the BBC Radio 4 programme *Today* and the BBC news.

Another way in which under-balancing was obvious was the use of journalists as sources.[3] Whilst the number of parents who had to make this vaccination decision were plentiful, journalists often used each other in order to represent public opinion. For example, on 10 February the *Observer* dedicated an 1,866-word article on the choices parents in its newsroom were making. Whilst the headline read "The MMR debate: PARENTS WEIGH UP THE ODDS", 18 parents were interviewed, all of whom worked at the *Observer*. The *Daily Mail* also ran a similar article on 6 February 2002, entitled 'THE GREAT MMR DILEMMA' where they reviewed the attitudes of 6 journalists, none of whom worked for the paper. Journalists account for 12% of all sources in broadsheets. Perhaps these examples are simply a sign of deadline pressures, but nonetheless, by selecting other journalists, they were guaranteed parents who are articulate and opinionated. This practice also illustrates journalists' tendency to use anecdotal evidence 'based on conversations with people similar to them' which, as Lewis and Wahl-Jorgensen argue, 'tells us more about the journalist's world view than what citizens actually think' (2005: 105).

Table 4.1 Balance of evidence presented

	Anti-argument only	Pro-argument only	Balanced
Mail on Sunday	64%	0%	36%
Sun	51%	14%	35%
Sunday Times	50%	8%	42%
News of the World	40%	30%	30%
Daily Mail	36%	7%	57%
Daily Telegraph	30%	17%	53%
Mirror	21%	49%	30%
Guardian	20%	26%	54%
Observer	13%	25%	63%
ITV early evening	13%	25%	63%
Today	13%	13%	73%
BBC early evening	0%	0%	100%

By examining the highest category for each media outlet (shaded boxes in Table 4.1) it is evident that, except for the *Mirror*, for each media outlet either anti-MMR or balanced stories were most common. The pattern of coverage suggested either an equal debate or stories emphasising the dangers of the MMR vaccine.

Balancing *Sources*

Vaccination statistics showed the vast majority of parents chose the MMR vaccine and by far the majority of scientists argued the vaccine was safe; nonetheless, most stories balanced sources in such a way that for every pro-MMR source there was an anti-MMR source. Almost half the sources (48%) spoke in support of the MMR and 38% spoke against and 14% were neutral or unclear. Placing sources in direct opposition to each other 'is a somewhat standardised feature of news reports designed to evoke sentiment and identification in human dramas' (Seale 2002: 142).

Analysing how media outlets balanced sources reveals the differing political motivations of different media outlets. Media outlets traditionally more sympathetic to the Labour government (*The Mirror, Observer, Guardian*) used more pro-MMR than anti-MMR sources, with three-quarters of all *Guardian* sources supporting the MMR vaccine. Predictably, right-wing newspapers (*Daily Mail, Mail on Sunday, Sunday Times*) selected more anti-MMR sources, or were more likely to have a more equal balance between pro- and anti-MMR sources (see Table 4.2). These statistics reveal the ability of newspapers to frame health and science stories in such politicised and biased ways.

Table 4.2 Source opinion on MMR vaccine by media outlet (n=643)

	Pro-MMR	Anti-MMR	Neutral
Mail on Sunday	19%	65%	16%
News of the World	40%	50%	10%
The Sun	40%	50%	10%
ITV news	42%	50%	8%
Sunday Times	41%	48%	11%
Today	34%	41%	24%
Daily Telegraph	36%	40%	24%
Daily Mail	35%	40%	26%
BBC news	43%	29%	29%
Observer	47%	31%	22%
The Mirror	56%	32%	13%
Guardian	74%	14%	12%

For a newspaper that has an anti-MMR and pro-single vaccine position, the *Daily Mail*'s selection of sources is interesting. There is only a 5% difference between the anti- and pro-MMR sources in the *Mail* articles and a quarter of all sources were either neutral or their opinion was unclear. As established in the previous section, the *Mail* used the discourse in articles to make accusations against the MMR vaccine rather than using direct quotes from sources.

Balancing Scientists and Health Professionals

Of the scientists and health professionals who were the first source in stories, 56% were anti-MMR vaccine; this did not reflect the views of the vast majority of the scientific community. The media more often chose to use scientists and health professionals whose views supported Wakefield and the anti-MMR lobby than the majority supporting the MMR vaccine.

Rarely were scientists presented or interviewed together; instead, they were more likely to be balanced with politicians or parents. Scientists balance each other in only 11% of the stories (see Figure 4.3).

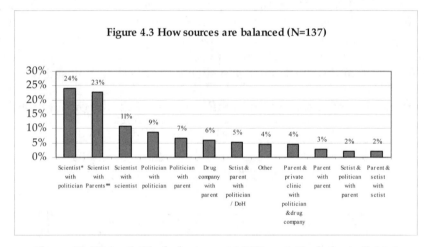

Figure 4.3: *'Scientist' includes 'experts', **'Parents' includes 'activists'.

In these articles, what most commonly occurs is Wakefield's research is juxtaposed against the bulk of the remaining scientific evidence or with a politician. The following *News of the World* article by Keith Gladis, deputy political editor, juxtaposes politics with science from the first sentence. When parents state they do not trust the MMR vaccine, it is politics and not science that they blame:

> TONY Blair has failed to convince parents that the MMR jab is safe, an exclusive *News of the World* poll reveals. Four out of ten people do NOT trust the combined vaccine against measles, mumps and rubella despite a massive campaign to reassure families. Our ICM poll reveals that the government faces a crisis of confidence over MMR. Just 60 per cent of people support the official view that the vaccine is safe and should be given to youngsters...Doubts about MMR began when it was claimed there could be a link between the vaccine and autism. Critics said parents should be given the choice of having separate jabs against each of the diseases on the NHS instead of the combined vaccine. The government refused to make separate vaccinations available—So many children were left with no protection against deadly measles...critic Dr Andrew Wakefield, whose research raised

safety concerns, said health chiefs were treating the public like a "moronic mass".

(*News of the World* 10 February 2002)

Previous findings about expertise conclude that 'reporters often seek experts who can represent each side of a controversy to present a more balanced picture of the particular scientific finding or claim' (Conrad 1999: 290). But this was not the case with MMR findings, as shown in Figure 4.3. Instead, what is clear is that journalists rarely balanced scientists with other scientists. The role of expertise and expert-sources in the MMR/autism story is examined more closely in Chapter 7.

Balancing Health Professionals and Parents

When pro-MMR health experts were sourced, balance was often provided by pitching these medical experts against parents. This created a serious difficulty for scientists and health professionals, who were often only able to offer dry generalisations and scientific evidence versus the more emotive and sympathetic figures of parents concerned for the welfare of their children. With most scientific experts lined up in support of the MMR vaccine, balance was often provided by pitching medical experts against parents and politicians, occurring in almost half (47%) of all stories. The role of parents in this balancing act allowed anecdotal evidence from parents with autistic children to enter the discussion—which, whilst not authoritative as scientific evidence, was powerful rhetorically. Few stories balance parents with parents, as in the following BBC piece:

> **James Westhead (journalist):** Little Benjamin's not having the MMR but three separate jabs. His mother Michelle Mcfadden-Jewer paid privately because she thought the MMR jab made her elder son Jacob ill. Now Health Secretary Alan Milburn is a family friend but there's been a serious falling out. Michelle says every parent should be allowed to choose the way their child is treated.
>
> **Michelle McFadden-Jewer:** Parents aren't ignorant, they've read the research and lots of people have gone against the government and is proved by the figures. So really I think it's about time now they said, fine let's use the single vaccines until there's proper research that's looked into it.
>
> **Westhead:** The private company that Michelle turned to has dealt with eight hundred families in the North East and says it has a huge waiting list but local health providers follow the government guidelines that individual jabs are not the answer but that the MMR is the safest way forward. And in the

end that's the choice June Dalton made for her daughter Kate, a series of measles outbreaks convinced her to go for the MMR.

June Dalton: It's the most difficult decision we had to make so far regarding the children's health. You feel guilty if you don't actually take them for it and then if something was to happen you would feel guilty for them having it.

Journalist: Are you glad you did?

June Dalton: Yes, we are now.

(*BBC* 28 March 2002)

Instead anti-MMR parents are more likely to be seen challenging pro-MMR scientists. The following piece, an excerpt from a piece over 6 minutes long, is typical of the coverage, using parents who rejected the MMR vaccine positioned opposite a scientist:

> **Dr Helen Bedford (Institute of Child Health):** We know that by giving single vaccines the coverage of immunisation would be reduced leaving individual children at risk of the diseases but also allowing the diseases to circulate in the population.
> **Sue Saville (journalist):** But some parents worried about MMR believe they should have an option for single doses.
> **Parent 1:** I think there's sufficient enough concern and uncertainty that I don't see any down side in giving them the single jab.
> **Parent 2:** There should be a choice between the triple and the single injections.

(*ITV* 6 February 2002)

Pro-MMR parents were rarely balanced with anti-MMR scientists. If journalists were being 'objective', then there would be similar numbers of stories with pro-MMR parents/anti-MMR scientists and anti-MMR parents and pro-MMR scientists—but this did not occur. In fact, journalists' deliberate choice when selecting parents is another example as to how the anti-MMR frame prevailed: parents in the media were much more likely to be anti- than pro-MMR. Two-thirds, 67%, of parental sources quoted in the media sample were vocally anti-MMR compared to only 20% who supported the vaccine (13% were un-stated/unclear).[4] This was most apparent on the BBC *Today* programme, where not one pro-MMR parent was sourced in the period studied. Journalists often sourced parents for their views on research even though the parents were unlikely to have read the research. So, for example, when a review of MMR research was published (Donald and Muthu 2002) *ITV* turned to parents for their views on this research. Importantly, only those parents attending single vaccine clinics were interviewed and journalists did not balance their views with parents who selected the MMR vaccine.

> **Harry Smith (journalist):** At this clinic in South London hundreds of parents pay so that their children can have separate jabs for measles, mumps and rubella because they don't trust the combined vaccine. None we spoke to was reassured by today's report.
>
> **(Parent 1):** *Even the so-called experts have conflicting reports: some say there is a risk some say there isn't.* So if there's doubt in their minds then there's going to be doubt in my mind.
>
> **(Parent 2):** Well I only heard it this morning just before I was going to come. *But there always seems to be some other research that balances that out.* So I think that if I had thought about it I probably still would've come.
>
> (emphasis added ITV news 12 June 2002)

What is noticeable in this example is that parents are making overt references to how journalists' practice of balancing their reports affects the public's consumption of evidence. In addition, the journalist makes no attempt to correct the misleading statements made by parents. The use of vox pops such as the above also illustrates how 'casual representations of public opinion are often slotted into news narratives to fit the news agenda' (Lewis and Wahl-Jorgensen 2005: 103). The dominant narrative, that the MMR vaccine might be dangerous because of a possible link to autism, meant that those vox pops that fit this narrative, anti-MMR parents, were used more often than pro-MMR parents. The focus groups picked up on this—that certain parents were more frequently appearing, with one parent stating a typical source in an MMR/autism story:

> 'tends to be the people who have suffered from it more than doctors and people.' (V3)

Balancing public opinion with scientific evidence is a method by which journalists take scientific stories out of the realm of science and make a more general story, therefore hoping to attract a larger audience. In interviews journalists spoke of having to choose from two types of sources: *emotional* sources (usually parents or JABS) and *rational* sources, usually scientists and politicians. This led to science being balanced with emotion as scientists were balanced with parents or politicians. Very few sources on the emotional side represented the pro-MMR side. To represent the rational, technical side of science, journalists most often turned to the Department of Health or scientists doing current research. Bar the DoH, the scientific argument was not consistently represented by any other group, organisation or individual. When considering what other pro-MMR scientific sources they could have contacted on this story, most journalists stated 'authors of scientific papers' or 'vaccination experts' as the key people they would approach. Other than Dr. Andrew Wakefield, the specialist correspondents, many of whom had covered this story since the 1998 press conference, were not able to name one other scientist. [5]

Sources' Views of Balance

In the MMR/autism story sources were acutely aware that journalists, particularly specialist health correspondents, did not agree with Wakefield's theories but nonetheless included his theories and sourced him because of their adherence to balance and commitment to objective reporting.

> Part of the journalistic training is to present a balanced story, one side versus the other, equal weight to both equals a balanced piece. Whereas the science on MMR is 99% plus in favour of MMR, less than 1% against and that's not presented. Giving equal weight to both is not balanced in terms of the weight of evidence.
>
> (Health communication PR)

So, even when sources dealt with journalists who were aware of the uneven evidence, they knew journalists would still balance pro-MMR arguments with claims from Wakefield, JABS or politicians campaigning against the MMR vaccine.

> The nature of the media (is) that if you've got a story, it's only fair to put across another side. The media must be seen to be fair and it's just unfortunate that the way that can come across to the public is that there's a fifty/fifty debate rather than a sort of ninety-nine versus one debate.
>
> (Health communication PR)

All of the pro-MMR sources agreed that the balance on this story was not considered necessary[6] and labelled the coverage as a 'failure of journalism' (science communication PR). Sources argued that balancing Wakefield's minority view with the rest of science was further exacerbated by balancing scientific pro-MMR sources with emotional anti-MMR sources (frequently the parents of autistic children). Scientists were well aware that their messages were dry and rational compared to the emotion of family traumas and therefore their scientific opinions and statements were less likely to receive substantial coverage. One source shows concern for the frustrations of the parents of autistic children but at the same time sees how the media use this to the disadvantage of the scientific argument:

> One of the most powerful media images during the whole thing was the television images of parents of autistic children—I had this beautiful baby, he had the MMR, now look at him. And here's the child behaving in all these familiar ways of disturbed autistic behaviour. Very, very powerful…the media obviously goes to a good image, a good story with anecdote and elevates the emotional or the irrational. It's very difficult for a white coat to compete with that parent and the whole level of irrationality is created around the whole thing.
>
> (Health professional)

The practice of equating scientists with parents frustrated many sources on the pro-MMR side of the debate. One source insisted that there are implications for expertise when the two sides are equally balanced as this:

> (e)levates their (parents of autistic children) judgement over scientific experts which in general creates very serious problems and in an area like this can undermine a whole area of immunisation policy.
>
> (Health professional)

Pro-MMR sources criticised journalists for not being concerned with the effects of balancing Wakefield's theories and making Wakefield appear more widely supported and thus more credible. Part of the reason why sources were so concerned about the coverage was that they regarded the media as having a powerful effect on the public. One spokesperson believed that the media were 'at the heart of' why the MMR controversy started whist another source argued:

> Each time the press latches on to it (MMR vaccine) more and more parents get worried about it inevitably…the problem is each time parents get worried, some children will not have the jab. And those who don't will be less protected than they would have been if they'd had it.
>
> (Royal College)

Journalists' Views of Balance

Interviews with journalists confirmed that balancing stories is still very much a strategic ritual for journalists. Many journalists did acknowledge the effect balancing had on the MMR/autism story but they saw this as an inevitable part of their professional values and failed to view balance as problematic or negative. Even though they may have been personally sceptical of Wakefield's theories, specialist health and science correspondents, like their general news counterparts, just as frequently balanced their stories (see Table 4.3).

Table 4.3 How different journalists balanced the story

How story was balanced	Health/science correspondents	General news correspondents
Balanced	65%	59%
Only anti-MMR reported (or only anti-MMR sources)	18%	26%
Only pro-MMR reported	17%	15%

Journalists regarded balance as a professional ethic and if it led to controversy, all the better, for this makes the story even more newsworthy.

> **TB:** In terms of the story, if you've got one scientist or a group of scientists saying one thing and you've got a larger group of scientists saying (something) contradictory do you feel it is adequate or appropriate to balance that story equally – so that each have equal space, equal weight in the story?
> **Journalist:** Yes, I think I genuinely try to do that.
> **TB:** You genuinely try to do that?
> **Journalist:** Yes, the (newspaper) is a very old fashioned place and we're very keen on balance here.
>
> (Health editor)

When pressed further and asked to comment directly on the disproportionate weight of evidence in the MMR research she rejected this would affect the way she reported this story.

> **TB:** Does it concern you at all that the amount of evidence is so clearly skewed, one side has so much more evidence?
> **Journalist:** Well that's an opinion and I don't have an opinion.
>
> (Health editor)

This raises an interesting point, if you take this comment to its logical conclusion, then a simple assessment of scientific evidence, that 99.9% of research says one thing, then this journalist regards this not as 'reality' but as an 'opinion'. This has implications when covering the statements of other 'maverick' scientists—if a scientist said water caused cancer, yet 99.9% of scientists said it did not, would this journalist give each claim equal weight? This statement is an example of how journalists' commitment to balance can have a considerable impact on how stories are framed and reported. When so few scientists support a claim, should journalists report these maverick claims; indeed, 'which scientific view should prevail?' (Reed 2001: 290). Other journalists conceded the issue of balance was complicated in this story. One journalist offered a way of trying to weight Wakefield's claims against the rest of science.

> How do you balance Wakefield against 99 million other doctors?...I mean you can't do that, it's absolutely impossible. If I interview Wakefield and show a 15 second sound-bite of him and then a 15 second sound-bite of (Chief Medical Officer) Liam Donaldson then viewers say, well there's arguments on both sides. But hang on a minute, there aren't two sides, you know, there are maybe 20 guys in the world and everybody else. You can't actually balance that. Personally I do it by not interviewing Wakefield...I've tried to get other reporters to do this, personal conversations cause it's the only way of doing it and trying to convince them...To try and put phrases in like 'there is a very small minority of doctors who believe MMR causes autism whereas the overwhelming majority of professional opinion is that it doesn't'...You have to try to get over the point that it is not a balanced debate, it's not two sides of a see-saw which are equally, finely balanced, it's not like that.
>
> (Science editor)

One journalist stated she did not 'find it difficult at all' when describing how to balance Wakefield against the rest of science, and her views were more common, and she simply abandoned balance.

> One has to come to some sort of conclusion about who's right and who's wrong on it otherwise it's impossible to write. You simply can't write both views with equal depth on every story.
>
> (Health editor)

Another journalist was also open about abandoning balanced reporting as they believed the link between the MMR vaccine and autism was fatuous.

> I believe that it is wrong to say that the MMR is linked at all with autism or Crohn's disease and that's why I won't write it. It's like saying I wouldn't say if you go out into the sun and get burnt you wouldn't get skin cancer, that's wrong. So I wouldn't write that.
>
> (Health editor)

Analysis on the two journalists above found they more frequently omitted anti-MMR arguments and sources.

In contrast, when a journalist from the *Today* programme was questioned as to why only anti-MMR parents were sourced, they responded defensively:

> I don't necessarily accept that point. I mean you'd have to go back and check through all the stuff if you're talking about — vox pops, going out and asking people whether they're concerned about MMR. I can't imagine that they were universally all on one side of the argument, not the kind of thing we'd sensibly do.
>
> (Science correspondent)

When Niall Dixon, former specialist correspondent for the *Today* programme (now chief executive of the health think tank The King's Fund), did a story for the *Today* programme and chose not to source the parents' group JABS he was reprimanded by then editor Rod Liddle. This story was well-known within the BBC as the two argued about balance during an email exchange. The BBC radio science correspondent interviewed for this research stated he was aware of the conversation but stated he 'wasn't there', and when questioned if there was a deliberate choice by the *Today* programme to select only anti-MMR parents he stated 'no'. When questioned further as to why no parents who chose to have the MMR vaccine appeared on the *Today* programme he stated:

> **Journalist:** It's the point isn't it? They're (pro-MMR parents) not campaigning at all.
> **TB:** I suppose to be fair, many of the parents on the *Today* programme weren't campaigners they were just average parents who were interviewed.
> **Journalist:** It's not average parents who were interviewed, it's the parents of autistic children in a debate about whether MMR has an influence on autism...
> **TB:** My point is that was it an editorial decision — you're saying no, this was just the way we were reporting the story. Which is basically what you're saying to me?
> **Journalist:** Yeah. It's very loaded though. What a strange question to ask, people who've got something to say about the subject rather than people who haven't!
>
> (Science correspondent)

The assumption here is that parents who chose the MMR vaccine *have nothing to say* and therefore were not a useful part of any balanced discussion. As will be seen in Chapter 8, focus group participants who chose the MMR vaccine did hold very strong opinions and wanted their views to appear in media coverage.

Journalists were aware that Wakefield's views were marginal within the scientific community but few disregarded balance. They were aware that balancing might make Wakefield's side more prominent and some of the specialist correspondents used linguistic techniques to demonstrate the two sides were not equal. But ultimately, they regarded the practice of providing two sides to a story as more important than faithfully representing the scientific evidence.

Audience Expectations of Balance

How the MMR/autism story was received is dealt with in detail in Chapter 8, but it is worth noting the impact balance had on this story's reception. Audiences are familiar with the journalistic tool of placing two sources or expert-sources on opposite sides; they expect and look for balanced stories, telling 'both sides' (see, for instance, Schudson 1978, Bourdieu 1996, Tuchman 1972, Lichtenberg 1996). When focus groups were asked what type of information they wanted about the MMR vaccine, they were quick to state they wanted 'balanced' information so that they would be able to 'make up their own minds'. When focus group participants tried to imagine the type of information they wanted, their responses were comparable across all focus groups:

- 'both sides' (Groups 1, 2, 3, 4)
- 'pros and cons' (Groups 1, 2)
- 'arguments for and against' (Groups 1, 2)
- 'positives and negatives' (Group 4)

Findings from the focus groups and national surveys demonstrate that presenting the MMR/autism story as balanced had a significant impact on public opinion and affected vaccination decisions. Whilst some media reports did point out that the weight of scientific evidence suggested the safety of MMR, this was not the overall impression created by the coverage. When focus groups were told of the modest amount of research supporting Wakefield and his findings they were surprised, confused and angry—although with who was less clear. Many felt that the media coverage suggested a much larger body of work and support for Wakefield's work. When one focus group estimated the amount of evidence Wakefield had and when told of the actual amount they reacted with surprise:

> **M4:** And his research was based on *two thousand people* or not even that?
> **TB:** Twelve.
> **M4:** Twelve — a lot less…
> **V7:** I'm gob-smacked that based on that research we are in this situation! I am really gob-smacked!…
> **TB:** You're all looking at me with quizzical eyes. I need to say this for the tape. (laughter)
> **M3:** I'm reeling a bit.
> **TB:** Why are you reeling?
> **M3:** Because of the number. I'm quite shocked that's all on such small numbers. I am. I am shocked.
> **TB:** Just shocked or anything else?
> **M3:** Well I would say I feel a little bit stupid really, I feel I've been completely washed along with the crowd.

This level of surprise was typical across the four focus groups, suggesting this style of she-said-he-said reporting does not encourage deep understandings but instead leaves the audience without knowing whether any solid evidence actually supports either of the claims. Corner and Richardson (1993) and Seale warn that balance in health stories makes complicated health stories 'appear more simple and certain than they really are' (2002: 64).

The national surveys confirmed the findings from the focus groups that balanced stories were influencing audience understandings. When asked about the scientific evidence two-thirds of survey respondents believed there was either equal evidence or that more evidence supported Wakefield. Only a quarter correctly stated that Wakefield's speculative claim was actually contradicted by most research (see Table 4.4).

Table 4.4 Which of the following statements is true?

	April (n=1035)	October (n=1037)
There is EQUAL evidence on both sides of the debate.	40%	53%
The weight of scientific evidence currently suggests NO link between MMR vaccine and autism. (correct)	30%	23%
The weight of scientific evidence currently suggests A link between MMR vaccine and autism.	25%	20%

Even when journalists stated the strength of evidence, what the audience seemed to hear was merely that there were two competing bodies of evidence.

Not only was the public confused about the amount of science supporting the link between the MMR vaccine and autism, but the national surveys revealed the public also overestimated how many parents were choosing single vaccines – fewer than one in six gave the correct response (see Table 4.5). This is unsurprising since the media more frequently chose to source parents who were not giving their children the MMR vaccine. At the time the surveys were held, the correct answer was 'Fallen by a smaller amount'.

Table 4.5 "The MMR vaccine was first used in the UK in 1988. Research published in 1998 caused the first controversies surrounding the vaccine. Since that time the number of children vaccinated with MMR has ...?"

	April	October
Fallen by half	20%	20%
Fallen by quarter	31%	26%
Fallen by a smaller amount (correct)	17%	15%
No significant change	6%	5%
Don't know	26%	34%

These findings suggest that people are not necessarily responding to the details of media content but to a simpler association in which the repetition of the theme of declining uptake led to an assumption overestimating that decline.

The impression created by the coverage of the MMR/autism story was that there were two equally conflicting sides for and against the MMR vaccine. By sides, this means equal scientific evidence and equal numbers of parents and scientists for and against the vaccine. Journalists frequently equally allocated time and space to Wakefield's claims and those of the rest of the scientific community. Failing to adequately weigh evidence led to stories that were over-balanced, which, as the MMR/autism story demonstrates, led to biased reporting and subsequently significantly influenced audience understandings. The practice of over-balancing both sources and evidence was a significant way in which the anti-MMR side was emphasised. Journalists might argue that they stated Wakefield's theories were poorly supported but the content analysis of television, radio and newspapers revealed that balance was often achieved by consistently putting the pro-MMR side on the defensive. In addition, anti- or neutral sources outnumbered pro-MMR sources and more anti-MMR scientists were quoted than pro-MMR. The impression that there were two equally conflicting sides and that by equating the research, made Wakefield's theories more credible and valid. This was also done by under-balancing stories, where journalists chose not to challenge his theories by including references to pro-MMR arguments.

This research raises a number of questions about the nature and significance of balance in journalism. Many journalists continue to regard 'balance' as a professional practice used to report stories. Achieving balance in a story is more than simply splitting stories down the middle and giving each side a fifty-fifty balance. Should journalists, particularly those who report science and health stories, consider different ways of reporting stories other than providing simple balanced stories? Should they always seek to provide a precise balanced story? By 2002 the established discourse in articles was for journalists to include both the idea that 'MMR was safe' and 'MMR might not be safe' in every story. But this practice can reduce journalism to a technical exercise (Glasser 1992), and as Malcolm argues, '(w)hat gives journalism its authenticity and vitality is the tension between the subject's blind self-absorption and the journalist's scepticism. Journalists who swallow the subject's account whole and publish it are not journalists but publicists' (1983: 144). The MMR/autism story demonstrates balanced stories are not always the most effective or honest way of reporting a story. An objective account of the MMR vaccine would not have been balanced, because in reality, the evidence was not balanced. Thus, the stories that were either pro-MMR or showed the weight of evidence which supported the MMR vaccine were more accurate representations of reality.

CHAPTER FIVE

Sources in the MMR/Autism Story

The relationship between sources and journalists has attracted a great deal of attention from media scholars, arguing sources do more than simply provide stories, quotes or information. Sources can initiate or thwart stories, set media agendas and influence how stories are reported and understood (see, for instance, Gans 1979, Gitlin 1985, Soley 1992, Miller et al. 1998, Ericson et al. 1989, Manning 2001, Palmer 2000). A source can have control over how a story is interpreted and develop this by making themselves 'part of an ongoing social debate...(p)ower over interpretation comes from the ability to influence whether an occurrence will even gain attention in the news media' (Berkowitz and TerKeurst 1999: 129).

Research consistently shows how news is dominated by the preferred meanings of *elite* sources and that journalists turn to sources they believe possess authority and responsibility (e.g., Gans 1979, Glasgow Media Group 1976, 1980, 1982). Ericson et al. go further and suggest 'news represents who are the authorised knowers and what are their authoritative versions of reality' (1989: 3). Traditionally official sources such as the government have an advantage over pressure groups and the public because journalists regard the government 'as a natural source of information and tend to accord it automatic access' (Cracknell 1993: 13). Elite sources wish to ensure they are the 'primary definers of policy issues in media discussions' (Franklin 1999: 28). Research that examines sources in science stories finds that scientific sources are generally considered credible, and as such, they are frequently able to secure favourable coverage (Miller 1999: 215). When journalists over-depend on elites as sources, elites' ideas and angles tend to dominate how stories are told. This is the basic argument behind Stuart Hall's *primary definers* thesis (Hall et al. 1978, see also Herman and Chomsky 1988, Soley 1992, Bishop 2001). Primary definers are those:

'regarded by journalists as authoritative sources, placed higher in a hierarchy of credibility than competing secondary definers, by virtue either of their position as political "representatives of the people" or because of their "recognised" knowledge as impartial experts'. (Hall in Manning 2001: 145)

Elite sources are not always so powerful, especially in risk stories where journalists adopt a different approach to sources. If journalists deem a story a risk story, they may then become more critical of official sources, concerned about their sources' motives and journalists are thus open to treating different positions as legitimate (Dunwoody and Peters in Kitzinger 1999a: 66).

Researchers differ as to who they think dominates the source-journalist relationship. Gans (1979) argues sources 'lead', whereas Berkowitz and TerKeurst describe the relationship as 'a clash between interpretive groups, with the source interpretation frequently winning out over that of the journalist' (1999: 129). Lupton and Mclean are clear who holds the upper hand in medical coverage:

The government, doctors and members of the legal system primarily define what constitutes news about doctors and health care. Even when news reporting is critical of individual doctors or the medical practice as a whole, media discourse tends to legitimate biomedicine and the medical doctors who practice it by representing them as the ultimate authorities, the agents of action, with patients as the recipients of their actions.

(1998: 956)

This chapter demonstrates various ways of analysing sources and finds that the sources selected and the way they were presented provides further evidence of how the anti-MMR argument was more prominent. There are 61 different categories of sources in this analysis and the specificity of these categories is necessary in order to provide a detailed assessment as to how the anti-MMR side came to be the dominant frame.

Analysing the selection of sources and how this shapes news is important as journalists mediate reality by selecting which stories to pursue, the sources to interview and which arguments to emphasise (Coleman 1995: 68).

Table 5.1 Source categories

Scientist – pro-MMR	Scientist anti-MMR	Scientist neutral
Doctor (not GP) – pro-MMR	Doctor (not GP) – anti-MMR	Doctor (not GP) - neutral
Dr Wakefield	Nurse	Health other
GP – pro-MMR	GP – anti-MMR	GP - neutral
Teacher/Headteacher/ Nurseries	Lawyers	Public
Parents – pro-MMR	Parents – anti-MMR	Parents - neutral
Mother – pro-MMR	Mothers – anti-MMR	Mothers - neutral
Fathers – pro-MMR	Fathers – anti-MMR	Fathers - neutral
Journalist – pro-MMR	Journalist – anti-MMR	Journalist - neutral
Tony Blair	Politician Labour	Politician Conservative
Politician Liberal Democrat	Politician other	JABS
National Autistic Society	Autism groups	Autism Action Association
Autism Research Centre	Autism Research Unit	Business
Drug Companies	Direct Health 2000 (single jabs provider)	Single jabs private other
Visceral	Department of Health	CMO Dr. Liam Donaldson
Deputy CMO Dr. Pat Troop	Dr. David Salisbury (DoH)	PHLS/HPA
JCVI	WHO	BMA
Royal College General Practitioners	Royal College of Nursing	Medical Research Council
Royal College Paediatrics and Child Health	Science Media Centre	Celebrity
Experts	Critics	Campaigners
Other (patients' groups, police)		

Sources Selected

In the coverage of the MMR/autism story, it is perhaps not surprising that scientists and health professionals are the most frequently selected sources. But scientific sources do not dominate and account for only 23% of all sources: three-quarters of all sources are not scientific or medical (see the first column in Table 5.2). Politicians and government personnel (primarily the Department of Health) were the second most likely sources used and represented 15% and 11% respectively of sources quoted. Parents account for 13% of sources and pressure groups 9%. Most pressure groups consisted of parents, so when pressure groups are added to parents, these two groups account for 22% of all sources and are the second most common source.

Table 5.2 Frequency of sources used

Source	Totals	First source	*Today*	TV	Tabloid	Broadsheet
Scientist/ Health prof.[1]	**23%**	29%	17%	39%	12%	9%
Politician	**15%**	15%	27%	24%	22%	22%
Parent	**13%**	15%	15%	20%	15%	14%
DoH	**11%**	9%	15%	0%	11%	8%
Pressure Groups	**9%**	7%	10%	0%	8%	13%
Medical /health organ.	**9%**	6%	10%	10%	10%	13%
Experts/ critics	**5%**	6%	0%	0%	7%	2%
Journalists	**5%**	4%	2%	0%	3%	12%
Other[2]	**4%**	4%	5%	7%	3%	6%
Private health/ Drug co.	**5%**	4%	0%	0%	8%	3%

There was a significant difference in the sources selected according to the medium. Table 5.2 illustrates that a wider range of sources appear in newspapers, including the Department of Health, pressure groups, journalists, experts, private health care companies and drug companies. However, none of these sources appear once in the television sample. Because of time restrictions, fewer sources appeared on television, so there was a smaller range of sources used. When pressed for space, as television news is, journalists selected sources who they believed to be the main sources in this story: scientists and health professionals, politicians and parents who represent 83% of all sources used in television news. Scientists were more frequently sourced on the television news, comprising 39% of sources on television, dropping to 9% in broadsheets. The use of scientists, health professionals and medical organisations as sources is the same in both tabloids and broadsheets; they account for 22% of sources, thus challenging the idea that the tabloids are dumbing down. Politicians were the most frequent source in newspapers and on radio. Politicians appear most frequently in stories about Leo Blair's vaccination status or the availability of single vaccines on the NHS. Conservative politicians like the Shadow Health Secretary Liam Fox and MP Julie Kirkbride blamed the Labour government for measles outbreaks and also highlighted the disparity of the government's stance on 'choice' in the NHS.[3] A short article in *The Sun* ends with a succinct quote from Kirkbride absolving Wakefield and science of any blame.

> Tory MP Julie Kirkbride—campaigning for the right to have three single shots —said: "This outbreak is the Government's fault."
>
> (*The Sun* 2 February 2002)

The order of sources is important in setting agendas and influencing understandings (Fairclough 2003: 53). Further evidence that the MMR/autism story was more political than medical is shown when looking at the first source; politicians were more likely than a representative of the DoH to be the first source (15% versus 9%). Table 5.2 also examines the first sources in each story. Scientists and their organisations were most frequently the first source, but it was anti-MMR scientists who were much more likely to be the first source, thus they were able to set the frame and challenge the science of the MMR vaccine (see Figure 5.1).

Whilst scientists and health professionals were the most frequent first source, parents and pressure groups are the first source almost just as frequently, in 26% of all stories. The *Today* programme often used Jackie Fletcher, the JABS spokesperson, as the first source. The

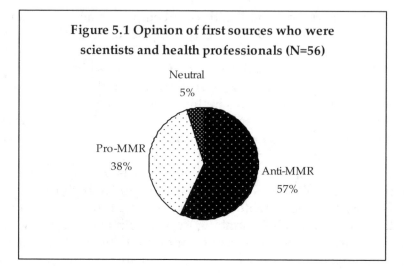

Figure 5.1 Opinion of first sources who were scientists and health professionals (N=56)

Neutral 5%

Pro-MMR 38%

Anti-MMR 57%

following story is typical; Fletcher, a vocal anti-MMR campaigner, with no science or medical qualifications, is the first source called upon to interpret newly published research. The deputy CMO Dr. Pat Troop is then put in a position to respond to Fletcher's accusations about the MMR vaccine.

> **Edward Sturton**: ....but it (Wakefield's research) came out on Panorama last night, hasn't been in a scientific journal yet, but Jackie Fletcher what did you make of it?
>
> **Jackie Fletcher:** Well again it's emphasising the need for research. We've got 1600 children believed to have been damaged by the MMR vaccine and up to date none of our families have been asked to give personal testimony and for these children to be examined.
>
> **Sturton:** When you say damaged by the vaccine, I mean, that's a supposition you're making, there's no clear evidence?
>
> **Fletcher:** Parents do believe their children have been damaged and the drug manufacturers actually specify these conditions in their own information sheets and most of the families are reporting problems in those drug sheets, just not at the one in a million rate that the bean counters are expecting.
>
> **Sturton:** But the fact is that however many studies, how many have been done, there has been no conclusive evidence about this link has there?
>
> **Fletcher:** Well there won't be until the senior medical advisors actually do a scientific study of the children believed to have been damaged.
>
> **Sturton:** Pat Troop, why don't you address that, what is the objection to that?
>
> (*Today* BBC radio 4 February 2002)

The published research is not discussed at all in the subsequent report except in the opening statement. The anchor, Edward Sturton, does challenge Fletcher's statements but then gives them legitimacy by using the same arguments to challenge the Deputy CMO. Fifteen percent of *all* sources were parents and when they appeared they were often able to frame the entire story. As two-thirds of parents sourced were anti-MMR, this meant 10% of *all* sources were parents choosing single vaccines or accusing the MMR vaccine of causing their child's autism. The following story is typical of those stories. Newspapers often placed these case studies alongside more factual articles. The entire text reads:

> JULIE Loch had no hesitation in allowing her 14-month-old son, Oliver, to be given the MMR vaccination. Her two older children, Matthew and Jessica, had received the triple jab and were both fit and well. But within weeks of being immunised, Oliver, who is now five, developed bowel problems and his behaviour changed dramatically. "Oliver was vaccinated in September 1997, and by that Christmas my husband and I were very concerned about his physical and mental health," said Mrs Loch, 37, who works as a part-time pharmacist near Cardiff. "Before the vaccine, he was a happy, cheerful and sociable little boy. People would comment on his big smile. But over the next weeks he became increasingly fractious. He started to have tantrums, scream and did not want to be held. Over the course of the year, he became increasingly more ill." Oliver was diagnosed as autistic just before his third birthday. He also suffers inflammation throughout his entire gastro-intestinal tract, for which he receives medication. There is no doubt in Mrs Loch's mind that her son's problems are linked with the MMR vaccination. "The only thing that changed was him receiving the jab," she said.
>
> (*Daily Telegraph* 7 February 2002)

In this case, not only does the parent set the tone for the discussion, she is the only source used: the pro-MMR side is not given space to respond to the parents' accusations. This is also an example of how logical science was pitted against emotional statements from parents. It also demonstrates why sources with emotional and anecdotal stories were valuable to journalists. Journalists argued the pro-MMR side needed to provide more vivid photo opportunities and more newsworthy sources. Many journalists interviewed did sympathise with the complex and difficult situation scientists were in but thought scientists could have done better.

> It's extremely difficult to say this to scientists: if you've got a very scientific case then in a way, certainly in a television report, you don't necessarily have to present the whole case. It's much more effective to show a kid brain-

damaged by rubella; that has much more effect than to show twenty scientists however important they are, saying "No, no, no MMR is alright". Because pictures speak to the heart, direct and don't go through the brain. And that's anathema to scientists you know, "we must make a rational decision", "people must have the information to make a rational decision' and of course they should, I'm not disputing that.

(Science editor)

Another journalist considered the efforts of the pro-MMR scientists and concluded:

They've presented as much evidence they could do, but they couldn't ever deal with the shear emotional side of it and the fact that Wakefield kept coming back and kept coming back and kept fighting his corner and giving his due.

(Health editor)

Most of the journalists interviewed also agreed that the pro-MMR message was difficult to promote and blamed the background and professional practices of scientists.

For tv, what you are actually showing people is emotion and that has an impact in a sound-bite and scientists don't do that, they're trained not to. They're trained to be factual, dispassionate, independent, fair, balanced and so on.

(Science editor)

The pro-MMR medical organisations will be discussed in more detail in the following chapter but it is worth noting how they are used in comparison with other sources. If individual scientists and health professionals were the most frequently appearing source, their medical organisations and professional bodies were much less significant, representing only 9% of all sources. When these scientific/medical groups did appear, it was often in a list of institutions that supported the MMR vaccine.

Controversy over MMR has grown despite backing for the triple jab from the World Health Organisation, the British Medical Association, the Royal College of Nursing, The Royal Colleges of Paediatricians and GPs, and the Community Practitioners and Health Visitors' Association.

(*Daily Mail* 7 February 2002)

Putting the MMR vaccine on the defensive was a much more newsworthy story, and therefore getting sources to accuse the vaccine of danger was more important to journalists:

The nature of the story was that they were always put into defensive mode and that's where they had to come from and also I think that at the end of the day, you know it's a big story, somebody questioning the safety of MMR is a much bigger story than somebody standing up and defending its safety and that's just the nature of news and the way the media works.

(Health communication PR)

Scientists more often appeared as individuals or as hospital doctors or GPs rather than as part of a wider, larger scientific community: any professional allegiance these scientists or health professionals held was rarely mentioned (see Table 5.3).

Table 5.3 Frequency medical and scientific organisations are directly quoted

Source	Frequency quoted
Public Health Laboratory Service/Health Protection Agency	22
British Medical Association	14
Medical Research Council	8
Royal College of Paediatrics	5
World Health Organisation	5
Royal College of Nursing	3
Royal College of GPs	2

The idea of a cohort of scientists or medical professionals supporting the MMR vaccine was rarely portrayed. This is important, as the idea of endorsement from a larger organisation adds weight to an individual's opinions: 'it is not just the personal prestige of individuals that makes influence so persuasive in social life; it is the credibility of institutions' (Mayhew 1997: 107).

Because the story had developed such a strong political frame, the main defenders/promoters of the MMR vaccine were not scientists but instead were politicians or representatives from the DoH. The following example typically turns to the government to communicate the benefits of MMR.

In an effort to combat...scepticism the government put up its Chief Medical officer to argue the benefits of MMR...The government is determined to get across its message about the benefits of MMR. But parents must still make up their own minds about what they believe is best for their children.

(Sue Saville, medical correspondent, *ITV* 7 February 2002)

Dr. Wakefield himself does not figure as often as his research find-ings; he is used as a direct source in only 19 of the 285 stories. He is discussed in 29% of main theme stories, but again, the difference be-tween media outlets is revealing. His name appears in 41% of broad-sheet stories, where there is physically more room to discuss background issues, compared to 25% in tabloid stories and 21% of television and radio stories (suggesting that this detail was an aspect of the story that was often dropped by those media with less space available). In addition, Wakefield appears more frequently in media that supports his own views. Fourteen of his 19 appearances occur in the *Mail on Sunday*, the *Daily Mail*, *The Sun*, the *Sunday Times* and the *Today* programme. He appears in a lengthy article in the *Sunday Times*, where the article's sympathetic tone gives him ample space to make his case.

> Wakefield, a former surgeon and consultant gastroenterologist, says the past few years have taken their toll. "I've lost my job, and my standing in the medical and scientific community is at an all-time low. There's no way I'm going to work again in this country. Nobody will want to employ me." He added: "What keeps me going is that I have to be able to face parents and say we did our best and we did not walk away from this because it was un-comfortable. And these parents at every stage so far have been shown to be right and therefore one is enormously reassured that this is the right course to pursue".
>
> (*Sunday Times* 10 February 2002)

As discussed in Chapter 1, Dr. Andrew Wakefield and his charity, Visceral, had access to the resources and skills of Bell Pottinger, a well-known and successful PR agency. Wakefield's practice of speak-ing only to those journalists who agreed with his theories was raised by a number of journalists as having a potentially powerful influence on how he himself and his theories were represented.

> I've actually had access to a lot of doctors and a lot of evidence and hearing Wakefield at the beginning, speaking to him occasionally, but he doesn't really want to speak to those of us who don't really agree with him.
>
> (Health editor)

Those journalists who agreed with his theories were often given ex-clusives to his unpublished research[4] and Wakefield's claims more frequently appeared in newspapers as this medium had the capacity to carry a wider range of sources.

TV's kind of different; you can always slide in a story on page 17 that's just a few hundred words, it keeps your contacts happy. But you can't do that on telly, you've either got to go big or you don't — so it's much more difficult to maintain that regular flow.

(Science editor)

Many sources were convinced that part of the reason why Wakefield received so much coverage was not down to the credibility of his research, but down to the efforts of his PR machinery, with a scientist stating:

'he's an arch publicist you know, he's got a very good PR machine available — *Private Eye*[5] and the lawyers who are promoting the MMR and the big American connection... in the right wing Republican party'.

(Scientist)

Why Wakefield or Visceral felt they had to resort to employing a PR agency is unclear, as neither Wakefield nor Bell Pottinger or Visceral will discuss this issue. Investigative journalist Brian Deer attempted to contact Wakefield via Bell Pottinger and after numerous emails with Abel Hadden from Bell Pottinger, Hadden admitted to Deer that he was not *employed* by Wakefield or Visceral, and conceded that he was working probono for Visceral. In my own interviews with sources they speculated that one of Visceral's board members was paying these costs. What we can assume is that with so many journalists supporting his cause, Wakefield and Visceral were well aware that the media played a significant role in securing public support and were willing to spend time fostering this relationship.

This research identifies the difficulty of using a term like 'official sources' because of the problem of defining who is an 'official source'. Are health professionals working in hospitals 'official sources'? Is Dr. Wakefield, as a scientist working at a hospital, an official source? Is he still an official source once he no longer works at the Royal Free Hospital? Health and science organisations and individuals were elite sources who provided expert knowledge – is this an 'official' comment though? The label 'official' is unhelpful in science, health and risk stories where it is unclear whether scientists are acting in an 'official' capacity or discussing research (whether funded by governments or elsewhere).

The Public

Research frequently discusses the powerful ability of elite sources to frame and define news but in the MMR/autism story lay voices played a crucial role. Whilst parents accounted for 13% of the total sources used, the use of personal stories had a significant impact. The emphasis on the 'average parent' and the effects on their families is a common convention used by journalists, especially in scientific stories. Brookes (2000) argues this in the coverage of the BSE crisis and Henderson and Kitzinger (1999) discover similar emphasis on 'dramatic personal accounts' in breast cancer coverage. Including lay voices can have 'a powerful effect' as they 'can offer a density that scientific abstraction cannot match' (Corner and Richardson 1993: 226).

Table 5.4 shows that the two television bulletins studied made more references to the public than newspapers or the *Today* programme. There is an escalating demand to include more 'ordinary people' in the news with television leading the way in this area (Hargreaves and Thomas 2002).

Table 5.4 Percentage of public as a source in all main theme stories

Medium	Percentage of all sources
Television	36%
Radio	16%
Newspapers	10%

Parents of children going for their vaccination, almost exclusively only those going for single vaccines, provided moving and candid sources. Their function was to discuss their emotions and their anxieties about the MMR vaccine. The stories parents provided were just too newsworthy for journalists to ignore, but this practice was criticised by some journalists.

> Anecdote is just incredibly strong and I think the newspapers ran with all those anecdotes whilst not running any of the things about the problems that measles could cause.
>
> (Science journalist)

> I just think there's been an awful lot of too, too lazy journalism...especially in the newspapers who've had endless interviews with parents who think they're kids are autistic because they've had the vaccine.
>
> (Science and health editor)

Part of the reason why so many parents were used as sources was because so many parents were willing to talk to them on this issue.

> It's such an emotional issue and it's not hard to get parents to give you emotional quotes on this one either, because they do feel very strongly, one way or the other, that they don't know what to do about it.
>
> (Health editor)

Kitzinger and Reilly argue it is important to analyse '(w)*hich* lay voice gains a hearing...and *how* they are presented' for these processes 'are far from democratic' (emphasis in original 1997: 347). The finding that two-thirds of the parents sourced were anti-MMR demonstrates just how important it is to specifically analyse which voices are heard. All parents of young children were having to decide whether or not to vaccinate with the MMR vaccine but journalists chose to represent only those who were against the MMR vaccine. The following BBC piece is representative, as it sources only anti-MMR parents and the only images seen are of those parents *not* choosing the MMR vaccine, but selecting single vaccines.

> **Parent:** It was the government who said it was safe to eat beef. Going back further I dare say there was a time when thalidomide was supposed to be safe. They have made mistakes in the past so I'm not completely convinced.
> **Fergus Walsh:** Isobel's mom isn't the only one who's worried. These parents were queuing up today at a private London clinic offering single vaccines at £60 a time. More than 8 out of 10 children are still having the MMR but a growing number of parents are prepared to pay for the separate jabs.
>
> (BBC 6 February 2002)

The way sources' views were presented demonstrated how certain lay voices were made more credible and influential. Journalists often let the vocal supporters of the MMR/autism link make claims without substantiation and elevated their allegations and authority. Author Nick Hornby wrote about parents who believed that the MMR/autism link was real and describes them in glowing terms.

> Let's assume there is a link between the MMR vaccine and autism. I know this is an enormous assumption, and that no such link has been proven (nor has it been disproven, despite Government suggestions to the contrary), but the point is that a significant percentage of parents with autistic children—*thoughtful, intelligent, observant people,* otherwise immune to conspiracy theories and paranoid delusions—are convinced this vaccine has irreparably damaged their children.
>
> (emphasis added, *The Observer* 10 February 2002)[6]

Part of the problem for the pro-MMR side was that it was easy to find parents with a strong opinion; journalists simply went to private clinics to source anti-MMR parents. Journalists could have just as easily gone to any GP practice to see parents having the MMR vaccine, but choose not to do so.

With so many parents willing to share their opinions and concerns with journalists, what did pressure groups offer that individual parents did not? Individual parents comprise 13% of all sources but journalists also turned to pressure groups, all anti-MMR, who made up 8% of sources. Both JABS and autism groups accounted for 8% of all sources, each at 4%. Parents and JABS were both portrayed as frustrated and worried with the developments of the MMR/autism story. JABS made more specific accusations and provided dramatic claims against the MMR vaccine than parents did. Pressure groups provided a human face in often dry scientific or health stories. Part of their power is in 'set(ting) agendas and defin(ing) issues when government or business refuse to talk to the media' (Miller and Reilly 1995: 318). Anderson demonstrates how Greenpeace did just this: they managed to define what was an environmental problem because the Department of Environment and scientists linked to these bodies 'did not act swiftly enough to "define" the problem' (1993: 64-65). JABS was eager and accommodating and all of the journalists interviewed had been in contact with them. JABS' key message was more newsworthy as they not only accused the vaccine, but also consistently criticised the government, as the following story shows.

> Jackie Fletcher, who founded Jabs and whose son has autism, says: "We have called on the Health Department time and again to carry out research into why these children's lives change so rapidly after receiving the vaccine. Even the information accompanying the combined vaccine points to adverse reactions. "It seems the Health Department has tried to panic parents into taking up MMR. But many are accessing the single vaccines — some travel to France where they are readily available," she says.
>
> (*Daily Telegraph* 25 June 2002)

JABS' role in the MMR controversy was twofold: to consistently provide parents who believed the MMR vaccine damaged their child and, secondly, to provide vocal support for Wakefield's views. When new research challenged Wakefield's theories they provided sources who supported Wakefield's position. Journalists labelled JABS as 'very helpful' (Health editor) and they 'played a very good game' (Science editor) and being 'very eager to offer parents' (Health editor).

Fletcher's media skills were demonstrated best on live radio, where she appeared more frequently than any other source on the *Today* programme. With the MMR vaccine consistently on the defensive, unsurprisingly JABS had few complaints about the coverage, even though almost all of their work comprised of responding to media questions.

> **TB:** Have you ever sent out press releases or statements?
> **JABS:** We have done sometimes, yes when there's been things going on, on the political side where perhaps we're inclined to get the Vaccine Damaged Patients Act changed. And there's things we've felt really needed to be in with a higher profile and we wanted to make sure it was there and sometime we have put press releases out.
> **TB:** What would be an example of say the last press release you went out?
> **JABS:** Oh gosh, that was a number of years ago now.
> **TB:** So you don't do it very often at all?
> **JABS:** We don't do it very often now because the media do tend to contact us at all times. (laughs)

There are other examples of small pressure groups being proactive and able to act as a powerful influence on how stories are framed and reported. In the coverage of AIDS in the UK in the 1990s, Miller et al. showed that resource-poor groups overcame their lack of financial and institutional resources by improving their media-relations skills (1998: 125). The Terrence Higgins Trust quickly established itself as an authoritative source for the media and successfully presented itself as a source of expert information and advocate for people with HIV/AIDS.

JABS had more influence than other pressure groups who supported the vaccine, such as the rubella charity Sense. The differing coverage between Sense and JABS again highlights the importance of examining *which* lay voices are used: JABS were sourced in 16 articles yet Sense did not appear once. The dangers of rubella or mumps were seldom discussed by journalists. On 8 February ITV science editor Lawrence McGinty met with a family who's adult child had rubella and was severely brain damaged. McGinty reflected on this piece and his observation that no other media outlet had discussed the dangers of rubella.

> We did do one piece that showed the consequences of not having vaccinations where we did a piece with a girl who's now about 18 who's brain damaged because her mother wasn't vaccinated against rubella...To be honest, I was proudest of getting that on than any piece I'd done that year because no one else had ever done that...We've got one piece a night and there's a mil-

lion other stories to do so I think getting that on was quite difficult. In a
newspaper it would've been easy.

(Lawrence McGinty)

Pressure groups promoting anti-MMR arguments received much
more coverage than those supporting it. But for a story dominated by
the fear of autism, autism groups and experts on autism did not figure significantly. The National Autistic Society's official line[7] was that
research pointed to the MMR being the safest way to protect children
against MMR but the NAS spokesperson sometimes went beyond this
message and argued single vaccines should be made available on the
NHS:

> As National Autistic Society spokeswoman Judith Barnard points out: "Par-
> ents have a right to protect their children. The government should make sin-
> gle vaccinations available on the NHS until research has been carried out."
>
> (*NOTW* 3 February 2002)

The remaining autism groups that appeared in the sample (Autism
Action Association, Autism Research Centre) are primarily research
based and all believe the link between the MMR vaccine and autism.
Coverage of these groups generally results from their attempts to
publicise their own research. There were no pro-MMR pressure
groups. Status quo pressure groups (comprised of the public and not
elites) are rare, for obvious reasons—if most of the public believes
what the pressure group believes, what's the point of the pressure
group?[8]

Labelling Sources

When labelling sources, linguistic practices made the anti-MMR side
appear more authoritative. Studying how journalists label groups and
individuals is important, for, as stated by Bell, in 'the media a title
embodies a person's claim to news value' (1991: 196, see also Matheson 2005: 24). Journalists used adjectives to make Wakefield's research
'more credible'. In three separate articles the *Daily Mail* refers to the
journal Wakefield published in as the 'respected' journal *Molecular
Pathology* (6,7,8 February 2002). When *The Sun* quotes the National
Autistic Society they are elevated to the 'the highly respected National Autistic Society' (*The Sun* 5 February 2002).

Anti-MMR parents were portrayed as making intelligent, thought-ful choices and were framed as the parents who were more worried. Parents choosing to have the single vaccines were labelled as worried more often than those who choose the MMR vaccine. It was as if the decision to have the triple vaccine was made by parents who were not worried and that worried/responsible parents, those who reflected on the decision, chose single vaccines. In *The Sun* a short article begins:

> WORRIED parents have clubbed together to organise their own clinic where kids can have three separate jabs instead of the MMR vaccine. Staff at pri-vately-run Direct Health 2000 told the anxious parents they would set up the kids' "outreach clinic" in Cornwall if more than 100 of them signed up.
>
> (*The Sun* 12 February 2002)

By constantly stating that anti-MMR parents were 'confused', 'frus-trated', 'increasingly choosing single vaccines', 'scared' or 'frightened' journalists chose to frame these parents in specific ways. In the fol-lowing article, the private clinic Direct Health 2000 mentions parents choosing single vaccines with respect.

> According to Kathryn Durnford, a spokesman for Health Direct, more than 15,000 children have been given a course of single jabs in the past 12 months. "We are now getting as many as 800 calls a day. These are *intelligent* parents, who feel that the present government policy of offering only the combined vaccination on the NHS does not give them a choice."
>
> (emphasis added, *Daily Telegraph* 5 February 2002)

It is in the interest of a private health care clinic to label their custom-ers as 'intelligent', thereby encouraging parents to believe if they se-lect single vaccines, they are 'intelligent'.

Private health care clinics account for only 3% of sources but they played an important role as they provided backdrops for journalists' pieces-to-camera and quick and easy access to anti-MMR parents. Like Dr. Wakefield, some of these clinics developed close relation-ships with certain journalists and media outlets. Direct Health 2000 was the only private health care provider directly quoted in the re-search sample and employed Dr. Wakefield after he left the Royal Free Hospital.[9] The fact that any of these sources might have a finan-cial stake in the outcome of the debate was seldom reported. Clinics and individual GPs offering single vaccines consistently spoke of the high demand, and few journalists challenged these claims or failed to state that most parents were vaccinating their children with the MMR vaccine.

Dr Peter Mansfield: By now the public has lost confidence in the situation and I'm afraid I think I see the end of the MMR policy looming. We are absolutely inundated with people wanting (the single vaccines).

(*ITV* News 6 February 2002)

Leading single vaccine supplier Direct Health 2000, a private clinic based in London, is using a national call centre with 200 operators to cope with demand. Spokesman Kathy Durnford said: "People are desperate for single jabs and we believe there should be a choice. It is clear that MMR is safe for a lot of children but we believe it is not safe for all".

(*Daily Mail* 5 March 2002)

It was in the interest of private clinics and physicians offering the single jabs to emphasise that their clinics were overwhelmed, setting the frame that there was a crisis and all parents were consumed with worry, and again, these statements went unchallenged.

Dr Richard Halvorsen: We are absolutely being overwhelmed, literally overwhelmed at the moment with enquiries for single vaccines. All the lines have been blocked all day and we've just had a crisis meeting now really in order to discuss how we can deal with this problem.

(*Today* BBC radio 7 February 2002)

Not one GP appeared in the entire media sample who stated they were busy vaccinating children with the MMR vaccine.

The majority of scientists and parents continued to support the MMR vaccine but the story's news values meant journalists often turned to anti-MMR sources to emphasise the idea of a controversy. Much research points to the power sources hold over journalists but sources are 'forced to accept the criteria of relevance that constitute newsworthiness in order to interest the journalist in the information' (Palmer 2000: 15). Sources have the potential to be powerful, but ultimately, journalists control what and who appears in the media.

There was a wide variety of pro-MMR sources for journalists to choose from: worried and vocal parents, scientists and health professionals, pressure groups, politicians and drug companies; however, these sources, with less news values, were selected less frequently. Thus, those sources which do not adapt their stories to meet the needs of journalists or make themselves newsworthy risk not being covered or their interpretation being ignored.

This chapter shows how the selection of sources and how they were labelled put the MMR vaccine on the defensive. In the following chapter, the activities and attitudes of health and science sources who supported the MMR vaccine are considered to examine their impact and influence on the MMR/autism story.

CHAPTER SIX

Behind the News – The Views of Health and Science Sources

This chapter examines the activities of the pro-MMR sources and establishes how their efforts, or lack thereof, also contributed to the anti-MMR side being a more dominant frame. Pro-MMR sources failed to set the agenda and spent a great deal of their time defending, and not promoting the vaccine. The health and science sources interviewed identified numerous difficulties in promoting the MMR vaccine, and when asked directly, some admitted defeat:

> **TB:** Who can represent the pro-MMR side?
> **Health communication PR:** ...There's no easy answer, I haven't got an easy answer, don't look at me, I haven't got a clue!

Journalists agreed that there were no simple answers as to what the pro-MMR side should do.

> **TB:** I mean if you're a scientist how do you battle against that?
> **Health editor:** (laughs) God knows, with great difficulty? I don't think there's an easy answer for it.

This chapter firstly considers the efforts of the main pro-MMR source, the Department of Health which was the principal promoter and defender of the MMR vaccine. This is followed by an examination of the efforts of other scientific bodies such as the Royal Colleges (for example, General Practitioners, Nurses, Children and Paediatrics), the British Medical Association, the Medical Research Council and the Science Media Centre. The chapter then considers why and how these sources failed to successfully challenge the anti-MMR discourse. Too often it is only the media who are 'blamed' for poor coverage or sensationalising stories. But as Miller argues, researchers need to consider 'the activities of the groups of actors and the interactions be-tween them that constitute the circuit of mass communication in rela-tion to science' (1999: 224, see also Gans 1979). The health and science sources interviewed had roles to play in the MMR/autism story but were unable or simply chose not to challenge media coverage. Were these groups correct in depending so much on the Department of Health to both promote the MMR vaccine and challenge its detrac-tors? Or should these sources have taken a more proactive and vocal role? This chapter examines their efforts and reasons behind their de-cisions.

Source Activity

The Department of Health

Sources and journalists had differing opinions on the role and efforts of the Department of Health in the MMR/autism story. The DoH ac-cepted they had full responsibility for arguing the pro-MMR message but stated they were not the only group responsible for this task. The scientific and medical organisations disagreed and argued promoting the MMR vaccine was not 'their responsibility' and that it was 'clearly the Department of Health's job'. Sources were 'sympathetic' to the difficulties facing the DoH and conceded the DoH achieved the best they could in these tough circumstances.

> I think they (DoH) handled it as well as they could. It is a difficult issue, it's an emotive issue, it's very difficult to explain and the public are naturally sceptical whenever the government says "don't worry, you know this is per-fectly safe". I don't have any complaints myself about the way the Depart-ment of Health handled it…They really are in a no-win situation.
>
> (Royal College)

> I think they had a classic scare story with all the right ingredients to go bal-listic but they worked with people which they're not always that good at. They have continued to hold the line on it…We'd be really quite annoyed if they didn't hold the line at this point.
>
> (Royal College)

These quotes might suggest sources were generally satisfied with the DoH, but the interviews revealed frustrations. Sources maintained that when the DoH was proactive, it did well, but overall, the DoH could have done more. One source suggested this would have been most effectively done with a 'discrete campaign involving the great, the good and the famous' (Health communication PR). Another source said the DoH was in an 'unenviable' position but they could have made more efforts and should have started defending and promoting the MMR vaccine earlier.

> They (DoH) were always on the backfoot and although they mounted a sort of public relations offensive eventually I think maybe if they had done that earlier, it might've been helpful...They didn't always put spokespeople up, sometimes they declined to comment and I'm not sure that that was right. I think it might've been better to always put somebody up but, generally I think they did the best that they could considering it was a crisis.
>
> (Health communication PR)

Most of the journalists interviewed rejected the idea that the media were alone to blame for the decline in the MMR vaccine uptake or the panic surrounding the vaccine. BBC science correspondent Pallab Gosh, when discussing media coverage of the MMR vaccine, asked for studies to be carried out 'into how the Department of Health and associated scientists dealt with the story' (2003) believing them to be partly responsible.

One reason why the DoH was not proactive and did very little was because they knew any statement they released would be balanced with an anti-MMR source, usually a statement from Wakefield or JABS.[1] As such, they made a deliberate decision to be less active so as not to provide more space and time for the anti-MMR proponents.[2] For the DoH, ideal coverage was no coverage. Their research established that any coverage, whether new research discounting Wakefield's theories or statements supporting the MMR vaccine, led to a decline in vaccination levels.

> Whenever there's coverage about MMR the coverage almost always mentions the "controversy", its links to autism, whether or not that's not the substance of the story — that is always mentioned. And that has an impact on parents' confidence, that has an impact on coverage. *So a great deal of the work that we do in the press is trying not to have any coverage.*
>
> (emphasis added, Government spokesperson)

The DoH acknowledged they were battling not just against scientists, but against campaigning media outlets less concerned with the scientific arguments and more preoccupied with scoring political blows against the Labour government.

Our tone didn't make a blind bit of difference to the coverage because people ignored what we said. I mean the difficulty was that what we were saying did not fit the story so it did not run…It's one of the difficult things in
terms of engaging at a scientific level and there isn't a debate, it's very hard
to work out what it is then that you're meant to say.

(Government spokesperson)

In trying to find out what the DoH was 'meant to say' the DoH involved 'all sorts of people' including civil servants, communication
personnel, scientific advisors and government ministers. Incorporat-
ing all of these views and trying to manage this range of contribu-
tions, would be difficult for any communications team. Add to this
the lack of trust in government sources and it was near impossible for
the DoH to have a consistent, coherent and effective communication
plan and successfully defend the MMR vaccine.

The efforts of the Department of Health divided journalists. The
journalists interviewed regarded the DoH as the main advocate of
vaccination policies and the defender of science but many were very
critical of the DoH's efforts. Journalists stated the DoH had only one
key message, that the MMR vaccine was the safest way to vaccinate
your child. Journalists claimed the DoH did little else to promote or
defend the triple jab besides consistently publicising this official
statement. The repetition of this key message bored journalists looking for newsworthy copy.

Well they have an absolute view and we do know they have an absolute
view and we expect them to come from that position. So the fact that they do
come from that position is kind of kind of no surprise to anybody…They got
a bit zealous really I think.

(Health editor)

Other journalists, because they agreed with the DoH on this issue,
were more sympathetic and thought the DoH did the best job it could.

I think Donaldson did an excellent job cause he was available…He made the
case as strongly as he could and he actually got fired up about it as well,
personally, he got fired up about it and a bit annoyed and a bit angry and
that helped. It actually helped to have the Chief Medical Officer saying, visi-
bly, not exactly losing his temper, but getting a bit shirty, because it shows a
depth of emotion. That's the problem, especially for TV, not so much for
print…What you want someone to say is to bang the table and say "look ba-
bies are going to bloody die because of this!"

(Science editor)

This emotional rhetoric was not welcomed by some journalists, who wanted scientists to remain dispassionate because, otherwise, the scientific evidence would become less important.

> These are the people who are supposed to say we'll come to you for the reasoned argument...the dispassionate verdict and actually you've got an agenda as much (as the parents). I think that's been quite influential in journalists' minds. I would say that they have found that they're getting a position being argued at them from the people they're going to for a more dispassionate overview and that has tended to increase cynicism.
>
> (Science correspondent)

The DoH rarely used the Chief Medical Officer Dr. Liam Donaldson, as their research showed he was not the most trustworthy source. As Donaldson was both a representative of government and science, this combination meant he was distrusted by parents and it was better for the DoH to recommend other, more neutral-appearing scientific experts.

> **Government spokesperson:** (The) basic research that we've got about who the public believe is that independent scientists are ten times more credible than government ministers, three times more credible than government scientists—which means we rarely will put up a Minister to talk about MMR, only really under duress. But either Pat Troop, the Deputy Chief Medical Officer or Liam, the Chief Medical Officer, rarely, Liam will do it once a year...We usually point the media at people that have done research into the safety of the vaccine like Helen Bedford, David Elliman, Liz Miller, Brent Taylor.
>
> **TB:** So the health and science correspondents would see them as independent?
>
> **Government spokesperson:** More independent than being people directly on the Department of Health's payroll.

The DoH was not abandoning scientific expertise when recommending other sources. In their published literature promoting the MMR vaccine, they continued to depend on and utilise scientific expertise and evidence. But parts of the scientific community criticised the DoH for doing so, for being 'incredibly arrogant', as an editorial in the *British Journal of General Practice* asserts:

> It is striking how many times (the DoH website) used the word 'expert', as if the use of this mantra will quash any disagreement. The DoH appears not to have noticed that experts are no longer instantly deferred to by the medical profession, let alone the public.
>
> (Jewell 2001: 876)

Journalists agreed and stated the emphasis on scientific expertise was characterised as didactic and insensitive to the emotional concerns of parents.

> I mean I can see what they're doing, "We're gonna get this through" and "We're gonna do it" and "We're just going to give people the science" and 'They are just going to have to understand, they're just being over-emotional'. But I just don't think that works anymore. You know I just don't believe that that works.
>
> (Newspaper columnist)

One of the key messages in promoting the MMR vaccine was to emphasise the dangers of measles, but these efforts were often criticised. GP Mike Fitzpatrick slated the DoH's use of the outbreaks in London and the North East of England hoping that they would learn that 'trying to counter one panic by promoting another panic is not an effective strategy' and that '(a)nxiety is not conducive to rational decision making' (2004: 37). Many parents over the age of 30 had experience of measles and used their personal experience to disparage the effectiveness of the DoH's messages.

> (The DoH was) somewhat dishonest about the whole business...in the sense of overstressing, the ghastliness of measles. You know it is awful but my sister had it really badly and I remember it very well...measles killed children before antibiotics. There's a whole load of stuff you can treat the symptoms with now. I mean, they go in for scare-mongering, they certainly do.
>
> (Broadsheet health editor)

When journalists offered advice to the DoH and pro-MMR scientists, most commonly it was to state they could have done more to challenge anti-MMR coverage or spoken with emotion, in a way parents would be more likely to listen to and value.

> There is a point at which the pro-lobby has to sort of take on those views and that language and explain to people...Talk back to people with metaphors that they can understand, in language they can understand. Instead of just saying no...I think all of this could've been prevented.
>
> (Newspaper columnist)

Other journalists argued that scientists took the wrong approach with journalists and were too overbearing.

> Perhaps treating people as grown ups and reasoning with them rather than sabotaging careers and launching attacks on individuals.
>
> (Science correspondent)

Opinions about the DoH's efforts were inconsistent. Sources and journalists criticised the DoH, but at the same time, they acknowledged the various pressures and influences on the DoH and understood the parameters they were forced to work within. In general, there was agreement that the DoH could have done better, but exactly how was less clear. There was agreement that the DoH was not capable of being the only promoter or defender of the MMR vaccine, nor was it the best. If both journalists and sources could see this, why did other health and science organisations not play a more significant role in the MMR/autism story? As the following section demonstrates, they were largely absent from the coverage and did not provide background information to journalists about the MMR/autism story.

Royal Colleges and Related Health Organisations

The role played by medical organisations such as the Royal Colleges or related medical bodies is seldom analysed in health and science stories. Karpf points to the reputation of the British Medical Association in the 1980s and that their pronouncements 'are widely reported, and fortified by their impeccable pedigree...most medical broadcasters pride themselves on their close association with the medical establishment – in Britain the Royal Colleges and teaching hospitals' (Karpf 1988: 111). However, whilst these organisations have an influential role in health, their public relations efforts are infrequently studied and little understood.

In interviews, sources from these organisations stated they felt powerless, arguing that the frames journalists used to report the MMR/autism story were entrenched against the DoH, i.e., government advice, that Wakefield's PR efforts were successfully influencing journalists and that emotional statements from parents were persistently more news than the views of rational science. So sources were aware they had a battle to change the dominant anti-MMR frame, but what was their most common strategy to try to challenge this coverage? To simply *respond* to media queries and *react* to what journalists asked of them. The following statement is typical of all the health and science sources interviewed. During an interview, one source from a Royal College dug out their log of phone calls from journalists over the previous year and a half and reflected as he looked at them:

> It's been largely reactive rather than proactive that's for sure. We have,
> we've been trying to inform, trying to restore a balance to the debate. What

you have there is more or less the sum total. I mean those three sheets of paper are more or less the sum total of what we put out publicly. We've spoken to journalists at least 12 times…It's not a major effort certainly.

(Royal College)

It comes as no surprise then that journalists are indifferent to the Royal Colleges, who represent thousands of doctors, nurses and midwives, or that journalists failed to regard them as key players in health and science stories. Each journalist interviewed was asked about the efforts of the Royal Colleges and one health editor admitted he 'can't remember ever using them very much' and another stated she knew little about the activities taken by them:

They haven't taken a view and anyway they haven't anything very interesting to say to be honest. You know, this is public health, it's not a matter, it's not a medical matter, not really…certainly I'm not aware of the Royal Colleges having looked at it.

(Health editor)

The desultory efforts of these organisations is best represented by the attitude of the Royal College of General Practitioners in responding to requests from the media to interview GPs. At this stage, the RCGP did not provide GPs for journalists to interview, arguing GPs are 'very busy' and instead suggested ways of getting in touch with GPs (often recommending journalists to get in touch with their own GP). The RCGP provided journalists with one spokesperson on the MMR/autism story, a vaccination expert. For journalists looking for GPs to source, the health professional most parents would turn to for advice, the RCGP was of little use. Only the British Medical Association offered GPs as sources. Not only did the RCGP not provide GPs for interview, they, along with many other Royal Colleges, willingly provided anti-MMR health professionals as sources, even though their official stance was that the MMR vaccine was the safest way to protect a child from measles, mumps and rubella. Thus these medical organisations provided sources both to defend the MMR vaccination programme and profess its safety and sources who argued the MMR should be given in three separate jabs or that the link between the MMR vaccine and autism was credible.

They (journalists) come to us for practices to visit and they will ask us, they will ring up, do you know a GP who is for, a GP who is against. We will supply them with a GP for and a GP against.

(Health communication PR)

Only one Royal College stated they would not put forward members who were against the MMR vaccine. They went on to state they would not criticise doctors who do not support the MMR vaccine, arguing that to do so was tantamount to censorship.

> We certainly don't criticise, we would never put out a statement criticising somebody with a different view because we don't. That's condemnation, that's not choice, that's not democracy.
>
> (Royal College)

The problem with not challenging doctors or health professionals from within their profession was that these anti-MMR statements often went unchallenged by the profession itself. In the media these anti-MMR GPs and scientists were able to challenge the safety of the MMR vaccine without any reaction from the scientific community because they believed it was their right, as scientists, to hold any view. Both the RCGP and the BMA believe it is the right of GPs to offer single vaccines and felt any derogatory comments were inappropriate.

The key messages of these medical organisations depended on scientific arguments and evidence. Many of the Royal Colleges stated their main message on the MMR/autism story was to 'represent their members'. The MMR vaccine was therefore regarded as a health issue; 'it wasn't a political issue from our point of view'. Instead sources labelled the MMR/autism story as 'a health concern'. For an issue that received such significant coverage, many sources admitted they did not have a 'key message' to promote and instead they were more likely to only *respond* to journalists' queries. As many of these sources were communicating similar messages—pointing to the amount of evidence supporting the safety of the MMR vaccine and the lack of evidence linking the vaccine and autism—they felt they were repeating the DoH's statements and therefore their views were redundant. The health and science sources believed that promoting and defending science was not necessarily what journalists wanted to hear and they made little efforts to challenge the dominant anti-MMR frame:

> I suppose what I'm trying to say was that was our role in (the MMR/autism story) was to defend the integrity of the science but that wasn't actually what the story was really about.
>
> (Health communication PR)

Most of the medical organisations' key message differed little from the DoH; some labelled it 'identical', and therefore, they felt they had little to add to the media coverage.

> The strength of the argument is almost that we and the Department of Health and the other medical Royal Colleges and the BMA are all basically saying the same thing, (the MMR/autism link) is an interesting idea, but the scientific proof really isn't there.
>
> (Royal College)

Did any of these sources try to make their arguments more newsworthy? Some of these organisations acknowledged that their complex and at times formal arguments were not effectively challenging the emotional claims of parents making the link between a child's autism and the MMR vaccine. As a result, some sources succumbed to media requests to make their stories more personal and shared their personal vaccination histories. These scientists and health professionals understood that personalisation is a necessary part of making research newsworthy and many of these science organisations now use personalisation to try and obtain coverage for themselves.[3] But others disagreed with this practice, stating that providing this human face ignored the science and was based on low expectations of the public.

> You're basically saying that the public cannot cope with a rational argument about the evidence unless they see the human victims...I don't really agree with that.
>
> (Science communication PR)

The Lancet editor Richard Horton agrees:

> The view that the public cannot interpret uncertainty indicates an old-fashioned paternalism at work...If one of the results of freedom of choice is an adverse outcome for the public's health, that is a regrettable but necessary consequence of our democracy. (2003: 214)

It is interesting that these two professionals dealing with the communication of scientific information hold the view that the public should be trusted to make their own decisions. For these two sources, providing more opportunities for science to make its case in the media results in the public being more able and more likely to make their own decisions. It is also in *The Lancet*'s interest to hold the view that the public wishes to inform themselves, because the public might then turn to them in order to educate themselves to make their own decisions. It is interesting that these two sources, who provide information to the public and patients, think so differently from those professional bodies like the Royal Colleges, who thought it best for the public to approach a health professional for the best advice. Their faith in the public to consume and retain knowledge is more optimistic than those organisations which deal with the public on a daily basis—as patients in their surgeries and hospitals.

Overall, these organisations representing thousands of doctors, nurses and health professionals were overlooked and not considered key sources by journalists on this important public health issue. This was partly down to their own lack of efforts. Despite being aware of the actions of Wakefield and other anti-MMR sources, they were no more proactive. All the scientific and medical organisations acknowledged the proactive character of the anti-MMR side in employing professional PR, using medical journals to improve their credibility and providing newsworthy material to journalists. Yet this awareness did not lead to these organisations becoming more proactive or making their own message more newsworthy.

Reasons Behind Source Activity

So on the whole, the medical organisations did not make great efforts to engage with the media, but *why* did they choose to make this decision? Sources offered a number of reasons why they were not more proactive; their reasons ranged from arguing it was a 'lost cause' as the frames were so well established, stating it was 'not their job', to maintaining that the most effective promotion of the triple jab was done outside the media. Some organisations, both supporters and challengers of the MMR vaccine, did little media work as they had few complaints about the coverage and therefore were not prompted to participate in media coverage.

Frames Too Difficult to Challenge and the Complexity of the Pro-MMR Argument

One key reason why so few pro-MMR sources offered stories to journalists was because they regarded any efforts as fruitless against the dominant anti-MMR frame. For example, sources who offered stories about children damaged by measles, mumps or rubella had little luck in securing coverage. Sense, the rubella charity, did offer stories involving severely disabled adult children affected by rubella, but as the media analysis showed, they received little coverage. When Sense was approached, it did not always go as planned:

> The *Daily Mirror* did a double page spread, went into Sense (which) set them up with three or four different mothers and their children…Everybody in Sense ran out the next day to buy the *Daily Mirror,* they'd seen the spread, they were sent it at the end of the day before with the pictures and the quotes. And instead (what) was (published) was "what celebrities think of MMR". They never ran it.
>
> (Science communication PR)

The rubella charity Sense believed journalists ignored them because their key message was the same as the DoH, endorsing the triple vaccine.

Another reason why pro-MMR sources felt unmotivated was because they could see the MMR/autism story was more political, about trust and governments, than about scientific arguments. The DoH spokesperson repeatedly stated the difficulty of promoting the MMR vaccine and asking parents to trust the science they had commissioned. The DoH admitted the MMR/autism story was more newsworthy when journalists applied a political frame and changing or challenging this frame was too difficult for them to do on their own.

> You know, (journalists) believe we're (DoH) lying, deceiving people and hiding the truth from them.
>
> (Government spokesperson)

Related to the entrenched anti-MMR frame and the difficulty of challenging them was the complexity of the pro-MMR argument compared to the simplicity of the anti-MMR 'it's not safe' argument. The health and science sources pointed to the complexity of the science, the difficulty of communicating that proving a negative is not possible (that MMR does not cause autism) and the difficulty in reducing their messages into media-friendly sound-bites. One journalist admitted that a fundamental problem for the pro-MMR argument was that 'anti-people always get more attention than pro-people' (Health editor). In their interview, JABS did not once mention that their anti-MMR claims—that the 'MMR vaccine causes autism', that 'MMR vaccine is unsafe' or that 'single vaccines are safer'—were difficult to communicate. Part of the problem was that the message 'MMR is the safest way to vaccinate your child against measles, mumps and rubella' takes some time to explain to journalists and parents.

It's very difficult to get across the message "we know this is not absolutely safe" (100% guarantee is not possible)...Now if you're not very careful the journalist cuts that to "MMR is not safe" full stop. To develop that argument in many media places is actually quite difficult. Given a long programme, that's fine, we can do it, we did do it...The reality of trying to get across that complex message is very, very difficult.

(Scientist)

The difficulty of making the pro-MMR argument in a short space or time meant that media coverage was more sympathetic to the simple messages of the opponents of the vaccine. Offit and Coffin outline the difficulties of defending the MMR vaccine in straightforward language:

Out of respect for the scientific method, aware of the fact that one cannot accept the null hypothesis, and mindful of the limits imposed by the size of epidemiological studies, we do not say "MMR vaccine does not cause autism". However, neither the media nor the public may understand the reasons for our reticence.

(2003: 4)

This complexity led to frustrations for those communicating the pro-MMR argument, who were dealing with journalists who often wanted uncomplicated and certain statements.

Certainly post-BSE, nothing is safe. Crossing the road isn't safe, getting on a train to come to work in the morning isn't described as being safe, nothing is a 100% safe. We've been using terminology like "safest" or "safer"...We never say something is 100% safe. But it still gets reported that we say "it's safe"...(Journalists ask) Why can't you guarantee to me that it's a 100% safe? Of course we can't within the bounds of scientific possibility.

(Government spokesperson)

The difficulty of understanding why science could not provide certainty or prove a negative was a frequent complaint by science and health sources.

It's difficult though to explain why the lack of evidence is so important, because no one is ever going to prove that MMR does not cause autism. You can only show that there is a decreasing probability that there is a link and there will always be that last half a percent chance that perhaps there is a link...Somebody said you could actually show a really good link between autism and shoes because, on the whole, autism shows up just about when you start putting children into shoes.

(Royal College)

As a result of the complexity of the science, some science and health sources were inhibited and discouraged from trying to make themselves more newsworthy.

'Not My Job'

Many of the sources who labelled the DoH's efforts as poor were also quick to give a reason why it was not their organisation's responsibility to promote or defend the MMR vaccine. They claimed they did not 'have the resources to make it a priority' (Royal College) whilst others stated it was not a priority for anyone but the DoH 'because we all had a day job to do and we all had other things to do' (Health communication PR). For the Royal Colleges, especially those with few or no press officers, they had to select the issues they could campaign on.

> For a long time our media policy was to keep as low a profile as we possibly could… we don't need people to know about us in order to do our job. Our job is basically overseeing postgraduate medical education…and even if no one in the country had heard of us…that would be fine…we've discussed this ad nauseum and think simply we need a high profile in certain circles, in professional circles, with ministers, with opinion formers but not necessarily with the public as a whole.
>
> (Royal College)

For these sources the MMR vaccine is just another medical story, and therefore they did not regard it with particularly high concern. That these sources did not regard the MMR/autism story as important to them was demonstrated by their failure to remember basic details of the coverage. When asked in interviews one year later as to why the MMR vaccine was a story in 2002, most interviewees could not remember why it suddenly hit the headlines. Most failed to remember the *Panorama* programme and Wakefield's publication in *Molecular Pathology*, which the documentary was based on. Many answered the question about why there was so much attention in 2002 with 'I haven't prepared' or 'I haven't done my homework' and one of the Royal College representatives could not remember Wakefield's name:

Royal College: The doc, who's name I can't remember.
TB: Wakefield.

With another unaware of the decline in MMR uptake:

> Do you actually have any figures on MMR uptake in 2002 as opposed to 2001? I actually haven't seen anything but then I wasn't really looking out for it.
>
> (Royal College)

At the same time as sources arguing it was not their responsibility, many took this one step further and stated they had 'no axe to grind' to 'defend' the vaccine or that they were neutral bystanders in this story.

> You know we have *no particular axe to grind* on anything. I mean certainly on MMR if decent advice, if decent evidence turned up tomorrow showing there was a link we would change our position immediately.
>
> (emphasis added, Royal College)

> I think broadly journalists have recognised that we *don't have an agenda* of our own here, that we are here to talk about the science to do reviews of the science to explain the science you know, whatever is needed. That we are independent and don't actually have an *axe to grind* as it were.
>
> (emphasis added, Health communication PR)

These sources were generally more concerned with their own organisation's messages and issues than with the MMR vaccine or the credibility of scientific research.

The idea that defending/promoting the MMR vaccine was 'not my job' was further exacerbated by structural or institutional constraints on some pro-MMR sources. The Medical Research Council openly admitted they could not be more proactive on this issue because their primary responsibility was to promote the scientific research they commission and not science in general. The MRC stated they were not responsible for defending the vaccine but for defending scientific research, and as their organisation had done little research in this area, they were reluctant to be used as a source. The BMA's structure also did not lend itself to proactive work promoting the safety of the MMR vaccine, as their primary role is to act as a union and to represent the views of doctors.

If organisations like these were reluctant to openly endorse or promote the MMR vaccine, it was then left to individual scientists to take time out of their schedules to defend the MMR vaccine. The scientists who did so usually worked for universities or medical schools. Physicians working for NHS trusts are not permitted to speak to the media without permission from their employer, hence very few hospital doctors were used as sources. As the Royal College of GPs chose not to provide GPs to journalists, journalists were left with a paucity of expert medical opinion advocating the MMR vaccine.

Because Dr. Wakefield and JABS had little, if any, structures to adhere to, they had more freedom to be proactive in promoting their own ideas and were able to more easily select the journalists and media outlets they wished to speak to.

Influence More Effective Outside the Media

Many sources avoided journalists because they claimed that the media distorted their key messages and that media coverage resulted in unwarranted attention to the MMR vaccine. They believed it was more effective to bypass the media altogether:

> I genuinely think doctors should be the ones who promote the message because all the evidence shows that they are the most trusted individuals of anybody…It's not for the Royal Colleges and the BMA, centrally, to say things. It is one million consultations that happen every day, that's where it should happen, in the surgery…The people who've read the *Daily Mail* then go to their surgery in the morning. It should be that GP who counters Lynda Lee Potter [4] cause I don't think anybody else can counter Lynda Lee Potter except the GP in their surgery with a young mum and her kids there.
>
> (Health communication PR)

> The bottom line is that the parent comes to the GP practice, they talk to the practice nurse, so you have a one-to-one with every single person who wants to talk about MMR and that's more effective use of your time than hoping that you reach people by doing a big media campaign.
>
> (Royal College)

A Royal College source stated that not one statement was issued, as they did not wish to escalate the story. Another explained the more they publicised the safety of the MMR vaccine:

> …the more people will suspect that there is a problem. You know 'the Department of Health commissioned this research and they're prepared to spend this money — surely, they must think there's a problem'. People stop having the vaccinations.
>
> (Royal College)

The DoH concentrated a great deal of their efforts on providing information to the health professionals who had direct access to parents making vaccination decisions. The DoH provided 'information direct to people and bypass(ed) the media', arguing the media 'doesn't ac-

curately reflect the information we want to get out'. During the research period, the DoH decided to abandon its large PR campaign to
promote the MMR vaccine in the media and instead decided to use
most of their budget and time working directly with health professionals (the campaign was named 'MMR: the facts'[5]).

This decision by the DoH and other sources not to actively promote the MMR vaccine meant that the majority of information journalists received was from anti-MMR sources, such as Wakefield and
other anti-MMR scientists. Thus there were few reasons for journalists
to write stories about the MMR vaccine that did not put the MMR
vaccine in a defensive frame.

Coverage Was Not Problematic

Some sources challenged the idea that media coverage was a problem,
arguing coverage was satisfactory and therefore they did not need to
do any pro-active media work. They pointed to the vaccination rates
as proof that coverage was not causing any great controversy or
health problems.

> I actually think vaccination rates are still quite high…but it's not like you've
> seen with something like GM food, where the consumer completely switches
> off and, and says I'm not eating GM food and supermarkets are forced to
> take it off their shelves. I mean that isn't actually what's happened.
>
> (Health communication PR)

Scientists from the Health Protection Agency argued that compared to
the pertussis vaccine controversy,[6] vaccination rates had not declined
significantly and concluded that 'the magnitude of the decline is small
and has been contained in the face of continued adverse publicity'
(Ramsay et al. 2002: 915). When asked to reflect on their efforts in this
debate, organisations were content with their effort and coverage.

> Your question was 'are you actually happy with it (the coverage of the MMR
> vaccine)' and I think the answer must almost certainly be 'yes' because we
> achieved almost exactly what we wanted to achieve. In other words, we got
> our message across when we needed to get our message across and at times
> we kept our heads down.
>
> (Royal Colleges)

Other sources claimed they played a significant role in the coverage,
but the content analysis found that none of the sources interviewed,
except for the DoH, were sourced regularly by journalists, nor did

their pro-MMR angle influence the media agenda. Interviews with journalists also demonstrated how little impact they had on how the MMR/autism story was reported. When sources listed the media outlets they believed were doing a satisfactory job reporting the MMR/autism story, they often omitted the more popular media outlets with high circulations, like the tabloids. A Royal College representative stated if 'you also read the *BMJ* and *The Lancet* and the medical press', the coverage would be more weighted to the balance of evidence in favour of the MMR vaccine. Of course, few members of the general public read these specialist publications and this naïve observation demonstrates how poorly some of the Royal Colleges and medical organisations were at understanding the public's needs.

Of those sources who argued coverage was not that problematic, many based this view on their own experience and on the number of media requests they had received. Very few sources carried out any analysis of the media coverage; most only collected stories about their own organisation or logged journalists' calls. For those sources who regarded the MMR/autism coverage was adequate, it was another reason not to do any proactive work to challenge the dominant anti-MMR frame.

Intimidation

Perhaps surprisingly, some sources indicated that there were attempts to intimidate and thus silence them. Wakefield often refers to the medical profession trying to silence him. *Lancet* editor Richard Horton described Wakefield as being publicly humiliated after the 1998 press conference, and he compares Wakefield to the scientist David Kelly, stating 'only those of a very robust constitution would have been able to stand up to the continued pressure of critics who wished to destroy his reputation' (2004a: 13). Horton emphasises this point by naming the section in his book on the MMR/autism story as the 'Malicious Reaction of Some Opponents' (ibid.). But those scientists who endorsed and promoted the MMR vaccine have also been at the receiving end of their own share of malicious behaviour. Dr. Brent Taylor of the Royal Free Hospital and other authors of scientific articles critical of Wakefield's theories have also been the 'targets of personal abuse by anti-MMR campaigners' (Fitzpatrick 2004: 36 and from personal interviews). The *Wall Street Journal* endured similar treatment when they published a column questioning Wakefield's science ('The Politics of Autism' 29 December 2003). A later editorial on 16 February 2004 ('Autism and Vaccines') stated they had received emails accusing the *Journal* of 'fraud' and being in collusion with the pharmaceutical industry. The editorial stated that their secretaries were 'harassed' with phone calls and one editorial writer was 'threatened' by a member of the public. Exactly who is behind these threats is less clear, but these examples underline the level of emotion on *both* sides of the argument.

Could Sources Have Done More?

What could pro-MMR sources have done to make themselves more newsworthy and secure better media coverage? Scientific sources, pro-MMR sources and sources promoting the status quo had a difficult time getting their message out because it contradicted what journalists considered newsworthy. Other sources believed they had little to contribute as their own views differed little from what the DoH was saying, thus they did not feel they were newsworthy. This raises two issues: even if all of these sources were saying the same thing and finding strength in numbers, they failed to take advantage of this unification and did not make use of the fact that non-government sources were more credible.

Of the organisations who agreed that coverage was a problem, few attempted to address the issue head-on, perhaps because there were no formal networks between the scientific and medical organisations. Some sources did admit that they wanted to do more proactive work on the MMR/autism story but they also admitted that the story did not change their working practice.

> We're still exactly where we were two years, five years ago, we react, we know what's happening, we know the statistics are likely to be awful, we know. We're not doing anything specifically for it. You're making me sound awful really.
>
> (Health communication PR)

What are the implications of the findings that many sources believed that the MMR/autism story was not their responsibility, coverage was not problematic or the frames too entrenched to challenge? The fact that the sources simply reacted to the emerging MMR debate rather than try to proactively become involved raised three key issues. Firstly, anti-MMR sources were able to set the agenda more frequently than the pro-MMR sources, who rarely, if ever, approached journalists with information or stories. When one source, the rubella charity Sense, did approach the media, they were deemed un-newsworthy by journalists, who were more interested in the scientific controversy and the risk of autism than with the risks associated with measles, mumps or rubella. Perhaps if more sources had made an effort to provide examples of the possible kinds of serious outcomes of these diseases, more attention might have been paid to this issue.

Secondly, sources must acknowledge they have less control over how the story was reported if they only react to journalists' queries instead of proactively working with the media. The RCGP's failure to provide GPs for journalists to interview meant journalists were free to interview or source any GP and begs the question: if the RCGP had provided GPs, would more pro-MMR GPs have been sourced? The efforts and influence of the Science Media Centre are also relevant to consider. The SMC was created by scientists who wanted to have more influence over the way science was reported in the UK media and one of their goals is to actively provide a wider pool of sources for journalists, as they did for the MMR/autism story.

> Rather than relying on the news editor of *The Times* thinking I need an opinion piece from a member of mainstream science, we offer them (scientists). So we gather together a group of scientists we know who are experts on MMR and we phone every news desk and say, MMR's in the news, who's covering it, we've got six scientists available today, who can do an interview. So we don't rely on the producers and journalists thinking of the right people we hand them to them on a plate.
>
> (SMC)

However, the SMC admits they were primarily 'reactive' when involved with the MMR/autism story rather than promoting the science. The SMC acknowledges they are 'proactively giving the media what they want. But in terms of who's setting the agenda, it's the media'. The head of the SMC goes so far as to state they were limited in the influence they had on how this science story was reported:

> Of all the debates about the way science is covered, this has been the one in which you can level the most criticism at the media.
>
> (SMC)

The final issue raised by sources' inactivity is that even when these sources knew rational arguments were not effective, they still depended on science to defend and promote the MMR vaccine. They acknowledged that the emotional and passionate arguments of parents were much more newsworthy than their own logical arguments. Only a few scientists discussed their own family's vaccination history to try to provide emotional arguments to counter these parents. If more scientists had adapted their statements to the needs of the media, then the pro-MMR argument would have been more newsworthy and easier to frame within the mainstream media.

What choice is there for sources if they cannot set the news agenda or influence how a story is reported? Was it worthwhile for pro-MMR sources to try to change the anti-MMR frame? The media were not discussing what the DoH and Royal Colleges wanted to debate, that is, the evidence pointing to the safety of the MMR vaccine, or Wakefield's inconclusive scientific research. But pro-MMR sources can be criticised for failing to organise news 'events' or altering their message so that it differs from the DoH in order to make themselves more newsworthy. Pro-MMR sources primarily depended on published research to make their case, but as the story was about more than science, they needed to provide events and information that were not just about science but that fit into the story's political frame.

Some pro-MMR sources agreed that their message did not get across as effectively as Wakefield's and they could have done more to promote and defend the MMR vaccine.

> Well in terms of the statutory duties, it's no one's job in particular—it might as well be us as anyone I guess again…but as you will have gathered I think the answer is eventually we have come round to the conclusion yes, it is us. Because nobody else seems to be doing precisely that job. Or precisely that job in precisely that way.
>
> (Royal College)

All the interviews took place in the summer of 2003 and a few sources stated that they would try to do more proactive work to promote the vaccine in the future. A public relations director at one of the Royal Colleges stated that the pro-MMR side 'needed more airtime'.

> …there are people who feel…that the message isn't getting over strongly and that something more proactive needs to be done rather than waiting to be asked on to talk about a study that says there's a measles outbreak and so on and so forth.
>
> (Royal College)

> The probability is by the middle of next year (2004) we will have done something on MMR but MMR is only one of a number of issues. I say obesity does actually seem to us to be the biggest issue of the moment.
>
> (Royal College)

By 2004 this Royal College had made the significant move to hire their first press officer. One scientist felt strongly that some organisation needed to do more:

> I think the Royal Colleges should take more of a role than they have...The Royal College of Paediatrics and Child Health for example, the Royal College of Physicians, the Royal College of Pathologists – there's a range of these are various expert bodies who I think must be trusted because they govern the whole structure of specialist health care in this country.
>
> (Scientist)

Another source agreed that one group or person needed to take control of the issue and that they wanted to take control, but they were too busy.

> It needed to be given to a group of people or a person, 100% of the time...There was a big flurry over one week or one fortnight and we suddenly realised, hang on, this thing is getting out of control. Now we didn't react to that cause we have other things on our mind no doubt, but somebody should've reacted immediately by maybe going to see editors to say, look, I know you've got to give space to this but do you realise what's happening?
>
> (Health communication PR)

One of the problems was that these organisations, the primary bodies representing doctors, paediatricians, GPs, nurses and medical research, did not meet or discuss their media strategies or the media coverage itself. Officials from these organisations often meet to discuss issues relevant to joint organisations in terms of policy or research, but they fail to discuss formally communication or media strategies. This is either done informally and infrequently between individuals and is not a structural commitment. A public relations manager from a Royal College admitted a network could have strengthened their message:

> I think if they are going to do something proactive they really need to get a number of organisations on board, we'd need to sort of link up with other people... A lot of people, a lot of GPs on an individual level are quite wor
>
> ried about the fact people haven't got faith in it (MMR vaccine) or believe in it.
>
> (Royal College)

As discussed in Chapter 1, in June 2006 scientists finally coordinated a response, albeit years after the controversy first appeared in the media. The SMC co-ordinated an open letter sent to the UK media and signed by 30 scientists. With the biggest measles outbreaks in the UK in 30 years, the letter asked journalists and the public to 'draw a line under the question of any association between the MMR vaccine and autism'. Appearing in a number of papers, the letter finally signalled a more proactive effort by these scientific organisations.

There is little argument over who represents the anti-MMR side: Wakefield and JABS were success in making these arguments and they were helped by campaigning media outlets and individual campaigning journalists. In contrast, the Department of Health held the main responsibility for promoting the vaccine and was the only obvious pro-MMR source. The pro-MMR sources interviewed agreed the DoH should have had help in relaying the pro-MMR message because of the declining trust in the government but they were not prepared to make substantial efforts to aid the DoH. The medical and scientific sources interviewed did not feel *responsible* for promoting the MMR vaccine. Some individual scientists were angry and did proactive media work because they were frustrated with the coverage, but they did not feel *responsible*. Perhaps the relevant question is not to ask who is responsible, as there is no disagreement here, but instead to ask a series of questions, resembling a simplistic PR plan:

- Is the story relevant to your organisation or your members?
- Will participation in the discussion affect your organisation or members?
- If yes to either of these questions, what are your key messages and plan of action. And if you decide to do nothing, how can this be justified?

Excluding Wakefield, most sources in the MMR/autism story were reactive; even JABS, who was very willing to speak to journalists, was primarily reactive. JABS was quick to provide emotional stories of exhausted and frustrated parents, give support to Wakefield's new publications, challenge pro-MMR research or criticise the government. Pro-MMR science organisations, like the Royal Colleges, were also reactive but provided little newsworthy material, and because the anti-MMR frame was set so strongly, they received little coverage.

CHAPTER SEVEN

Expertise

In an expanding media universe, with escalating coverage of health and science issues, questions of who to trust to provide expert information and opinion is a vital issue for journalists, academics and the public. Given this expanding media sphere it logically follows that more sources will be sought as more news is produced. How are journalists to understand which sources possess expertise and which simply have information? This chapter[1] uses specific categories of expertise—the Contributory-Interactional-None theory of expertise offered by Collins and Evans[2] (2002). The CIN theory provides a more coherent and consistent method of assessing and understanding expertise. Cottle identified the importance of analysing 'how exactly the "expert" becomes constituted and signified within certain milieux, including those of the mass media' (1998: 15). The division of expertise into a defined category, 'expert-source', separates experts from other sources who do not possess expertise. A more detailed definition of 'expertise' provides journalists with tools to make sense of what can seem like an overwhelming amount of information, what Seale labels 'a chronic flow of available knowledge' (2002: 14). A theory of expertise for journalists and academics offers a coherent method of deciphering a source's expertise. This chapter demonstrates how journalists used expert-sources and their claims in the MMR/autism story and how the representation of their expertise influenced the way the story was reported and received.

Expertise and Journalism

Many researchers have observed the paradox of the declining trust of experts; for example, Horlick-Jones (2004: 108) argues the 'chronic sensitivity to risk issues' results in a 'corresponding erosion of trust in sources of expertise'. But at the same time as this increasing dependence on expertise in Western society, '(w)e believe less and less in experts...(but) we use them more and more' (Limoges 1993: 424). Identifying the relationship between the use of experts by journalists and the decline in these experts and journalism is less well understood. The move away from a positivist scientific paradigm to one with 'less rigorous distinctions between scientific and other judgements' (Albaek et al. 2003: 939) can be attributed to the expanding range of topics on which someone becomes an expert. This shifting understanding of expertise translates into a volatile definition as more and more people consider themselves, and are regarded by others, as experts. Risk theorist Ulrich Beck sees this wider understanding of expertise as beneficial to societies which have elevated the views of experts (particularly scientific experts) during times of crisis and important national and international debates. Beck believes broad understandings of expertise free the public 'from (the) patronising cognitive dictates of experts' (1992: 168) and empowers the public to:

> (s)elect within and between expert groups...Not only are practitioners and politicians able to choose between expert groups, but those groups can also be played off against each other within and between disciplines, and in this way the autonomy of customers is increased.
>
> (ibid.: 173)

Beck views experts 'playing off each other' as beneficial to democracy, but in doing so he fails to acknowledge the potentially detrimental effects of this, such as confusing or frustrating the public and therefore decreasing the trust in expertise. Instead, Beck deems this cacophony of experts as an opportunity for the public to become experts themselves.

The role of expert-sources in the media and their effect on audience understandings is less well understood. The research which does exist falls into two categories: analysing *why* journalists select expert-sources and *how* journalists use expert-sources. Journalists select expert-sources for three main reasons: to provide facts, to add credibility and to present objectivity. Most commonly, expert-sources are used by journalists to verify and provide facts. For this reason, expert-sources may not appear in every story but they are an integral part of a journalist's working life, frequently providing background information (Levi 2001: 12, see also Conrad 1999: 291, Croteau and Hoynes 1994: 67). Credibility is another principal reason why expert-sources are selected. Manning argues that '(t)he possession of expertise helps news sources to rise up the hierarchy of credibility in the eyes of journalists and helps to ensure that they become regular points of contact on specialist correspondents' beats' (2001: 158).

Journalists also try to use expert-sources to enhance objectivity, but as Steele admits, in reality they 'often have decidedly partisan or political perspectives that are not acknowledged' (1995: 803). Expert-sources often regard their own expertise as neutral and become frustrated with journalists' need to balance what they (the experts) think is a definitive statement. At the same time as believing expert-sources provide 'neutral' comments, journalists also turn to expert-sources to provide opinions. Albaek et al. (2003) argue what journalists want from expert-sources has evolved. In the 1960s experts were more likely to discuss their own research, whereas from the 1980s onwards, they were more likely to comment on general social issues.

Steele's (1995) study of two daily American television news magazines, *Nightline* and the public television programme *MacNeil-Lehrer NewsHour*, examines how expertise is assessed. Steele concludes journalists had an ambiguous understanding of expertise and their use of experts was based on experts 'real world experience, access to and knowledge of the "players"' (1995: 805). She also adds the willingness of experts to 'make predictions' influences how journalists use experts (1995: 805).

The credentials of an expert-source is the most important influence on why certain expert-sources are selected. Van Dijk argues the 'media tend to use "experts" whose reputations and qualifications add weight to the argument being made, influence the way events are interpreted, and set the agenda for future debate' (in Rowe et al. 2004: 161). At times, it is not just any qualification but the right kind of qualification that is relevant; '(w)hile younger scientists are often most willing to talk with reporters, experts with recognisable names, titles, or affiliations are prized sources. The journalistic ethos suggests that a source should be a '"top guy (sic) in the field" to safeguard credibility' (Conrad 1999: 291). With this emphasis on qualifications, it necessarily follows that those expert-sources without conventional qualifications will be overlooked. Eliasoph (1998) uncovered situations where citizens, who had educated themselves and possessed a level of expertise, were not 'presented as knowledgeable'. She argues fault lies with both the public, who emphasise their emotions when talking to journalists and with journalists, who relegate citizens' comments 'to overly narrow, passionate, devalued professions of self-interest' (1998: 217, see also Miller and Riechert 2000: 51). Croteau and Hoynes' analysis of the American news programme *Nightline* also showed that those without 'appropriate credentials' were 'generally not worthy of consideration' and even when the public was lucky enough to participate in these discussions '(t)he interpretations that are highlighted, then, are not those of the public, but of the pundits who put it all into perspective' (1994: 59). There is the risk that the public, regardless of knowledge or expertise, will be regarded simply as emotional and not knowledgeable. This way of representing the audience, presenting only opinion and reaction and not knowledge, is typical in media representations of the public (Lewis et al. 2005).

Previous academic studies that analyse the use of experts in the media generally fail to define expertise or provide explanation of the significance or difference of expert-sources compared to non-expert-sources. For example, Croteau and Hoynes found *Nightline* used a 'litany of "experts" who were primarily ex-officials, most holding conservative views (1994: 177-178). Croteau and Hoynes did not ana-lyse whether these sources were experts or are simply elite sources with inside information (see also Anke et al. 1994, who come to a similar conclusion but also failed to define the source's expertise).

Research more frequently examines the *numbers* of experts in the news and not more what makes a source an expert. For instance, Al-baek et al. (2003) provide a detailed assessment of the increasing use of experts in their study of Danish newspapers over a 40 year period. They found a rise in the use of experts, explaining the increase was down to the increasing dependence on experts in wider society, the media's tendency to concentrate more on the needs of consumers and, lastly, the changing role in which experts interact with the society (Albaek 2003). Simply counting the selection of experts in stories can demonstrate society's increasing dependence on experts; however, this type of research fails to analyse levels of expertise and whether the experts presented are genuine experts and, consequently, the im-plications if they are not. The creation of an expert-source category, situated in a normative theory of expertise, seeks to provide research-ers and journalists with a way of categorising and better understand-ing expertise and expert-source selection.

'Expert-Sources': A New Category

In media studies research, sources are traditionally categorised according to status, the types of information they possess and/or access to information. These categories are not based on knowledge or expertise. The categories 'official/non-official', 'resource-poor' and 're-source-rich' relate to the *status* of an organisation or individual. The categories of 'official' and 'non-official' sources have been found to be restrictive and inadequate (see, for instance, Miller et al. 1998) and the MMR/autism story demonstrates the difficulty of dividing sources according to their official status. For example, should scientists working for universities be labelled differently from those working for governments or business? How do organisations like the medical Royal Colleges fit into these definitions? Source categories according to the *status* of the source are not specific enough to prove useful if analysing stories where expertise is inherent to the story, as is often the case in science, health and risk stories.

The categories 'primary and secondary definers', 'insiders/outsiders', 'arbiter and advocate' refer to the *type* of information a source can offer. Over time, sources move in and out of these categories. In the MMR/autism story, the parent led group 'Justice, Awareness and Basic Support' (JABS) were on the 'inside' in 1998, taking part in talks with the Labour junior health minister and the Department of Health but they were later ostracised from official processes.

Deacon and Golding's (1994) 'advocate' and 'arbiter' categories deal with the *activities* of the sources and not their knowledge. In the MMR/autism story all sources could be labelled as 'advocates' (holding of a point of view, e.g., scientists, the ruling Labour government, parents) but it is unclear who acted as the 'arbiters', those sources who assess the views of protagonists in a debate. 'Resource-poor' and 'resource-rich' categories (Goldenberg 1975) are also problematic due to the increasing use of public relations. PR skills help to level out those who are 'resource-poor' and 'resource-rich' as more and more organisations are aware of how to make themselves and their views newsworthy.

If considering the expertise a source possesses as a way of dividing and defining sources, it is necessary to have a coherent definition of expertise to differentiate between *sources* and *expert-sources*. Collins and Evans (2002) created a normative theory of expertise with distinct categories. They wished to preserve scientific and technical expertise, arguing expertise is central to our notion of how our society works. Collins and Evans divide expertise into three categories: 'contributory', 'interactional' and 'none' (CIN). This chapter argues expert-sources are those sources which possess specialised knowledge and encourage journalists and academics to consider expert-sources as either possessing contributory or interactional expertise.

The highest level of expertise is *contributory expertise.* This is the ability to contribute to an esoteric specialism and can be learned only through practice and total immersion in a subject. Contributory experts are able to *contribute* to the core set of knowledge in a specialism. *Interactional expertise* is mastered through linguistic socialisation alone and requires extensive immersion into the culture of a particular specialism. Interactional expertise is acquired through *linguistic engagement* with contributory experts. That these two categories state expertise is 'real' leads to the last category, which is having *no expertise.* The transition between no expertise and interactional expertise is accomplished by reading technical material, by *talking* to the contributory experts. The basis for Collins and Evans' criticism of contemporary definitions of expertise is the idea of 'lay expertise'. In Collins and Evans' definition there is no such thing as lay expertise, either you have expertise or you do not – whether or not you are a lay person (without credentials) is irrelevant.

Collins and Evans' definitions are closely related to experience; their contributory-interactional-none theory (CIN) moves from 'a discourse of trust' to a 'discourse of expertise'. The CIN theory believes experience is central to expertise and that without experience you cannot have expertise. But *experience cannot be a sufficient criterion of expertise.* This is a key point when discussing expertise and journalism – that experience is mistaken for expertise is common in journalism. For example, raising a child and observing their health does not make one an expert in child health. Yes, parents have the *experience* of numerous childhood diseases (and they may contribute to the core set of knowledge if they develop sufficient knowledge) but this does not mean that their statements are expert statements or that importantly in this case study, their views are not equivalent to expert statements. This balancing act will prove to have a significant influence on how expertise is received.

The CIN theory of expertise does not profess to solve debates *between* experts; instead it provides distinct categories of expertise. In the case of debates between experts, the CIN definitions provide normative categories to define who are the contributory experts, the interactional experts and who has no expertise. For instance, in the MMR/autism story more attention could have been paid to the lack of contributory experts in autism in the media coverage. It should be emphasised that the CIN definition of expertise does not argue that contributory experts are the best or only sources to turn to or the most valid form of expertise. Instead what the CIN theory offers is the idea that 'real' expertise exists and that not all knowledge is expert knowledge.

Which Expert-Sources Appeared?

Analysing the selection of sources used in MMR/autism stories reveals that sources were not necessarily selected for their expertise or knowledge in the area of vaccinations or autism. In the media research sample, scientific expert-sources did not dominate, with scientists accounting for only a third of all sources. Chapter 5 showed that just over a third, 37%, of sources were non-experts (politicians, parents and representatives from pressure groups). Whilst the most frequent first source were scientists and health professionals this only occurred in less than a third of the stories. Chapter 5 also demonstrated that the sources who appeared first, often framing the debate, were non-experts challenging scientific expertise. Whether or not pressure groups like JABS or parents had the expertise or knowledge to make their accusations against the MMR vaccine or any discussion of their level of expertise/knowledge was absent in media coverage and in interviews with journalists. Cottle might argue these parents are not presented as experts but are the 'ordinary voices' who embody and symbolise a subjectivist epistemology, an experiential way of knowing, feeling, sensing or 'being' in the world (2000: 37). However JABS and other anti-MMR parents were not presented as 'ordinary voices' but were often juxtaposed with scientific experts who were put into the position of answering parents' claims that the MMR had caused their child's autism.

In each of the three reports on the *Today* programme which JABS founder Jackie Fletcher, she is the first source to speak and scientists then respond to her claims. In the following piece discussing newly published research, which is just over six minutes long, Fletcher speaks for almost 3 minutes attacking the safety of the MMR vaccine.

Fletcher openly admits she has not read the research under discussion and instead uses her appearance on the *Today* programme to publicise JABS' key messages and fails to respond to the research. Fletcher is presented as able to assess the credibility of the research even though she has not read it – nor does she have any medical/scientific background or training.[3] Instead, she has the experience of raising her autistic child and her belief that the autism was caused by the MMR vaccine. The anchor, Sue McGregor, does not challenge Fletcher on her unsubstantiated accusations, but instead uses the accusations to challenge the scientist from the Medical Research Council:

> **Sue McGregor:** Jackie Fletcher we're in the realms of supposition now, if this new research, to be put up on the website today of the British Medical Journal, says more reassuring words about the triple jab would you be prepared to have a look at it?
>
> **Jackie Fletcher:** *I would be interested to see it.* What concerns me though is that we've got a huge body of children, we've got about 1600 believed to have been affected by the MMR vaccine and they've not been investigated by the Medical Research Council....
>
> **McGregor:** Well Dr. Peter Dukes is here with me. You know Jackie Fletcher and others believe the research hasn't really been good in this country to support the generally accepted theory about MMR.
>
> (*Today* BBC radio 8 February 2002)

The journalist used the claims of a non-expert to challenge the expert – and the claims of the non-expert are based on supposition, not on scientific data. If using traditional definitions of sources, Fletcher can be labelled as a primary definer or resource-rich (she has access to numerous parents who claim their child's autism is *caused* by the MMR vaccine). She is both an advocate and an arbiter; however, none of these terms give a sense of the impact of her views on the wider story. Considering the expertise Fletcher does or does not possess and then comparing this to scientists who author and publish research is a more useful way to understand why the MMR/autism story was reported in the way it was and how the anti-MMR frame became so dominant. The *Today* programme is less concerned with the expertise of Jackie Fletcher and is more concerned with the likelihood of Fletcher making sweeping and newsworthy accusations. As Palmer (2000) points out, a source's perceived news value also affects source selection and, in this instance, Fletcher's news value supersedes any notion of her possession of expertise. The editor of *The Lancet*, Richard Horton, picks up on the idea of who has the right to participate and set the parameters in medical debates:

Who are deemed to be acceptable public adversaries worthy of opposing one another? In the case of the MMR vaccine, the Department of Health, for example, has put too little emphasis on understanding the concerns and views of families with children who have autism. Are those families ruled out as non-expert and therefore inferior protagonists by our politicians and public health officials? If so, why?

(Horton 2004a: 44)

The families of autistic children possess experience in caring for their children who have a debilitating disorder, but this experience does not make them experts *in the causes of the disorder*. Are they therefore *inferior protagonists,* to use Horton's language? This is a disingenuous question because it does not follow that because they are not experts, they are therefore 'inferior protagonists'. That parents do not possess expertise does not make them 'inferior'. Parents' views can and should, still be heard, but their *opinion* should be regarded or presented as such, *opinions* and not equated with expert assessment.

In addition to analysing which sources or expert-sources journalists choose, it is also necessary to analyse what journalists choose to quote from these people and how this is presented. In reporting the MMR vaccine, journalists choose to mention single vaccines in 58% of all articles. This emphasis on single vaccines, as recommended by Dr. Wakefield, was seen as the only alternative to the 'controversial' MMR vaccine. In the following ITV report, a GP and well-known opponent of the MMR vaccine, argues for single vaccines:

> **Sue Saville (Journalist):** This GP provides single vaccines privately for parents who are worried about MMR.
> **Dr Peter Mansfield:** By now the public has lost confidence in the situation and I'm afraid I think I see the end of the MMR policy. We are absolutely inundated with people wanting to go otherwise.
> **Saville:** So why are single vaccines not available? The NHS does not supply single jabs because the government believe that MMR is more efficient, more effective and reduces the exposure risk to children.
>
> (6 February 2002)

This emphasis on single vaccines saw *The Sun* make recommendations of their own, based on no obvious expertise:

> *The Sun* has been demanding separate jabs for measles, mumps and rubella be made available on the NHS. Campaigners say single shots are safer than the triple jab — although the Government insists they can be MORE dangerous.
>
> (7 February 2002)

The Sun makes no appeal to scientific evidence or expertise but instead frames its advice in political terms. The single vaccines are to be trusted because of 'campaigners' and the MMR vaccine to be mistrusted because the government supports it. Expert opinion was dismissed in favour of political guidance.

Personal Opinion of Scientists

By 2002, the MMR/autism story had become one about government policy or parental confidence rather than the science of the safety of the MMR vaccine. The point is reinforced where we see even expert knowledge being put to the test in terms of the way scientists would treat their own children. Expertise is no longer trusted unless it can be seen to be validated by a willingness on the part of the experts to put their views into practice. The following *Daily Mail* article stresses not what scientists *know* but what they would *do*. The only remark that the scientist is allowed to make is *verbatim*, the most authoritative kind of statement, and is about how he would treat his own children if he had them:

> The new report was compiled by public health experts Dr Anna Donald and Dr Vivek Muthu of health study analysts Bazian Ltd for the British Medical Journal publication Clinical Evidence. They say they found strong evidence that both MMR and single measles vaccinations virtually eliminate the risk of measles and protect against mumps and rubella which themselves cause serious complications, including death. They found consistent evidence that MMR and single measles vaccines are associated with small, similar risks of fever within three weeks of vaccination. However, they point out that measles itself causes acute fever in all infected children. Dr Muthu said: "I don't have children, but if I did, I would not hesitate to give them MMR."
>
> (*Daily Mail* 13 June 2002)

Textual analysis shows that even when expert-sources were used, they often referred to their own experiences about making vaccination choices for their children. Here child health expert Dr. Helen Bedford writes in *The Sun*:

> As a mother of two young boys I understand how concerned and frightened some parents must be feeling about the MMR vaccine. No parent wants to take any risk with their child. Both my boys, aged six and nine, have had two doses of MMR and if I had to take them to be immunised tomorrow I would.
>
> (*The Sun* 7 February 2002)

Participants in focus groups stated they wanted to know the personal decisions of experts and found stories such as the above very helpful. The consequence of experts using reasons other than their own expertise is that their scientific evidence can become less important and less newsworthy than their personal statements. In addition, if scientists with children are using their own choice of vaccination as the reason why they should be trusted, conversely those scientists without children face the possibility of being ignored because they do not have children. *Daily Mail* columnist Quentin Letts picks up this point:

> The Chief Medical Officer, Liam Donaldson, does not list any children in the current edition of "Who's Who". Nor does one of the more strident pro-MMR politicians, Dr. Evan Harris of the Lib Dems.
>
> (*Daily Mail* 1 July 2002)

Levi writes that '(b)oth experts' *opinions* and scientific *findings* are relevant in medical stories. Both should be reported. However, they are not interchangeable' (2001: 59). But on this issue, journalists and scientists did, at times, swap expert-sources' opinions and findings. In interviews, scientists revealed they were under pressure to give personal opinions and some expressed their reluctance to turn to this personalisation of scientific evidence. Most were happy to share their personal experience in order to circumvent the complex scientific evidence.

Journalists were also required to provide personal opinions. Interviews with journalists found some had been asked by their editors to provide personal accounts of their own vaccination decision. Whilst it is the job of columnists to hold strong opinions and share them with their readers, this is not normally required of journalists. There is danger in confusing these two roles, in asking journalists to drift from reporting to commentating as seen in the following article written by the *Sun's* medical correspondent, Jacqui Thorton. Thorton normally writes news articles but here she writes candidly about her opinion on the MMR vaccine:

> Just over a year ago I wrote an article backing MMR, based on scientific research. I am still NOT convinced there is a definite link with autism, a condition which is said to affect 500,000 people in the UK. But throughout the last year, the Government has been so rigid, so unfeeling and so categoric on this issue that they have lost a lot of ground with parents who normally analyse the facts and make their own decisions. Now parents aren't prepared to trust the facts so often quoted by ministers. They don't want to take the risk. No

matter that hundreds of thousands of children have had the MMR and are perfectly okay.

(*The Sun* 5 February 2002)

Thorton's expertise as a journalist masks her lack of expertise in science. She chooses to make recommendations on the MMR vaccine in terms of *politics* and not science. She chooses to ignore the advice of expert-sources and chooses not to present their side in her article.

Balancing and Expertise

As discussed in earlier chapters, journalists choose sources and expert-sources for a number of reasons but they are often selected simply to balance a story, thus making it appear 'objective'. As established in Chapter 4, balancing non-experts with experts gives the non-experts a rhetoric of expertise in two ways, either through over-balancing (non-experts with expert-sources) or under-balancing (presenting one side of an argument). If an expert-source cannot be found to provide balance, then journalists can, and do, elevate sources to expert-source status in order to provide this balance. As a result, sources and expert-sources appear interchangeable. Into this confusing world of expert-sources and sources masquerading as expert-sources steps the media pundit. Seemingly available to speak on anything to anyone at anytime, pundits make expertise irrelevant. Journalists also play their part in the increasing use of pundits by elevating topics supposedly worthy of expertise. For example, psychologist Petra Boynton was asked to 'predict a man's sexual performance by his preferences in takeaway food', which she declined to do. When later reading the article she discovered the journalist had found an 'expert' who was able to make a connection between kebab-eating men and their sexual abilities. She states that 'too often 'expert' stands for 'the first person we found who would talk to the press, and who would say what we or our editor wanted to hear' (Boynton 2002). This is not simply the fault of journalists, but the fault of sources willing to comment or manipulate their own expertise to suit the needs of a journalist.

Journalists require sources who can provide quotes quickly. Bourdieu states television rewards those who are 'fast thinkers, who offer cultural "fast food" – predigested and prethought culture' (1996: 29). These fast thinkers, available any time of day and providing a lifeline for 24-hour news, are the numerous pundits employed by a variety of organisations, think tanks and pressure groups (for the rise of punditocracy see Soley 1992, 1994 and Hallin 1992). The rise in pundits allows journalists to explore opinions instead of facts:

> (P)undits are the people anointed by the media to give their opinion on things...Whether these people can be expected to bring any special expertise to their subject matter is wholly at the discretion of those doing the anointing. The ability to call oneself an 'expert' on a particular topic is useful, but hardly necessary qualification.
>
> (Alterman 1992: 5)

Alterman believes the 'roots of punditocracy can be found in the rise of objective journalism' and the 'demise of opinionated journalism' (1992: 304-305).

Chapter 4 found that 48% of stories were more likely to be balanced but in only 11% of stories are scientists balanced with each other (see Figure 4.3, page 82). In the majority of stories, scientists were balanced with non-experts – parents or politicians. In more than a quarter of stories, 28%, scientific sources were not part of how a story was balanced. Thus the majority of balanced stories used sources without contributory expertise, so the balanced debates lacked scientific evidence and instead used other types of reason, such as the political argument for choice between the triple and single vaccines. When members of the public are placed directly opposite experts, the public then 'become(s) accustomed to making critical comparisons between their own experiences and expert knowledge, to seeing ordinary experiences being accorded time and respect, and to seeing experts in conflict both with each other and with the lay public' (Livingstone and Lunt 1994: 99). By leaving these non-expert claims unchallenged the reader is left to make up their own mind, having heard only one part of the argument and from sources without expertise whose claims are often based on suppositions and intuition, such as the following from columnist Robert Harris in the *Daily Telegraph*:

> They (parents) have certainly produced no absolute scientific proof of their suspicions. Instead there are just a few scraps of disputed evidence, in particular a disproportionately high incidence of the measles virus lodged in the intestines of autistic children who have had the MMR vaccine. That— and the sheer, unscientific common sense which whispers in the ear of every parent: that to inject three live viruses into a baby certainly sounds like the sort of intervention that might conceivably produce, in a tiny fraction of cases, a catastrophic reaction.
>
> (*Daily Telegraph* 5 February 2002)

Selecting Expert-Sources

In interviews conducted for this research, journalists were reluctant to differentiate between how they selected sources and expert-sources. Journalists stated they did not use different methods to select expert-sources and non-expert-sources. Experts were simply a 'source'. One tabloid health editor argued she chose the expert-sources she 'could get hold of'. Journalists rarely discussed the expertise possessed by their sources. They argued assessing the level of expertise in a source was simply a matter of 'checking', of 'using their news sense' (broadsheet health editor). When questioned as to which pro-MMR scientific sources they would contact on this story, most journalists stated 'authors of scientific papers' or 'vaccination experts' as the key people they would approach. When questioned further, these specialist correspondents, most of whom had covered this story since 1998, were not able to name another relevant scientific expert other than Dr. Wakefield. Instead they named who they believed were the most relevant sources such as Dr. Wakefield, the DoH and parents. For journalists, possessing expertise was not as important as possessing newsworthiness.

To compound the complexity of journalists choosing which expert-sources to use in this story was the fact that some expert-sources purposely did not construct themselves as expert-sources. Many avoided doing so believing that the distrust of experts in society would mean that the public would trust them less or that journalists would be less likely to use them if they were regarded as experts. As a result of this declining trust in expertise and with the ghost of BSE still visible, many sources questioned whether to even bother making an effort to comment on this story.

> We were very conscious around all this time of the backlash against the establishment and we were very conscious of adding to it by entering the field … on this one (the backlash) was pronounced where there was a view that the establishment were all singing from the same hymn-sheet and therefore we didn't push ourselves too much.
>
> (Health communication PR)

That there were problems with the reporting of expertise might be explained by the training journalists receive. With more than a third of journalists in the UK now holding a qualification (Journalism Training Forum 2002: 36), journalism textbooks can perhaps provide some understanding as to how they consider expertise. On the whole, journalism textbooks dispense ambiguous advice to student journalists; find the best expert, ensure they are articulate and if they are not, find someone else. Sheridan Burns states that after an interview journalists need to decide 'whether to believe what he or she has been told' but offers no advice how to do this (2002: 81). The *Reuters Handbook for Journalists* says nothing about experts; its section on sources simply tells journalists how to correctly label them (MacDowell 1992). Mencher's book *News Reporting and Writing* is one of the few journalism textbooks to deal specifically with experts and he warns journalists to 'be careful to use sources only within their areas of expert knowledge' because a 'reporter's best sources are those who have demonstrated their knowledge and competence as accurate observers, interpreters and forecasters of events' (1997: 312). But as journalists often write stories about issues they themselves are not experts on, Mencher's advice is problematic.

The contributory-interactional-none categories of expertise aim to provide journalists and academics with a coherent way of asking sources how their expertise relates to a particular story. To reiterate, science/health stories should *not* only be composed of expert-sources with scientific backgrounds. Some science stories should be and are framed and reported within wider social contexts. By being more forthright about the expertise a source possesses, journalists can limit the influence of powerful or elite sources and potentially redefine the role of public relations, calling for their profession to provide sources with more specific and relevant expertise and knowledge.

Journalists already have strategies that encourage them to select sources which have a specialty in the field. This is not an argument that expert-sources are the 'correct' sources to use, but that journalists can be more open and forthright when using expert-sources. Journalists' contacts might now read along the lines of 'scientist', 'social worker', 'planner' but by using more specific categories of expertise, instead they will have more specific contacts such as 'physicist', 'biologist', 'social worker working with underprivileged children' or 'social worker working with ethnic minorities'.

The CIN definitions do not abandon the concept of 'lay expertise' but instead argue expertise is expertise—regardless of whether or not the subject is a lay person or a professional. The public's participation in a debate and their knowledge acquired through their lives make elements of a story newsworthy but their opinions or experiences should not be mistaken for or presented as expertise. Collins and Evans argue experience is key when analysing expertise.

> ...experience is central to expertise. Without experience you cannot have expertise. Experience is a *necessary* condition of expertise. But experience cannot be a *sufficient* criterion of expertise or anyone could be an expert in anything
>
> (emphasis in original, Collins and Evans 2007)

The effect of experience on expertise can best be explained by referring to Brian Wynne's (1989) well-known study of the relationship between Cumbrian sheep farmers and the UK Ministry of Agriculture, Fisheries and Food scientists after radioactive fallout from Chernobyl contaminated their pastures. Wynne established that these local farmers, with no formal qualifications, had 'lay expertise' in sheep ecology which the government scientists should have taken into account. The term 'lay expertise' has subsequently been picked up by bureaucrats and academics alike but it has often been re-interpreted as the expertise of lay people and used to emphasise lay perspectives rather than defend the use of expertise. Wynne's thesis led to a raft of projects celebrating the 'lay expert' and the corollary was often that scientific expertise was problematic.

CIN categories argue that the public has experiences in their *own* illness but are not experts in the illness itself (the public is capable of becoming interactional or contributory experts, as Epstein (1999) shows this occurred in the early HIV/AIDS crisis, but this infrequently happens). It is important to draw boundaries around the public's expertise, or lack thereof, because the media 'have increasingly come to construct the responses of ordinary people towards illness as authoritative and admirable, exploiting the fall of professional hero' (Seale 2002: 185). As such, certain lay voices have powerful news values, and '(s)ome "lay voices" have greater power and appeal than others' (Kitzinger and Reilly 1997: 347).

The CIN theory intends to expand the idea of expertise at the same time as setting limits or boundaries. The creation of categories will not prevent future disagreements between experts, but will seek to establish less vague debates and the use of more specific experts. Admittedly, some debates exist because experts cannot decide which experts are relevant. These definitions will not prevent debates but put more definitive boundaries around the use of expert-sources in these debates. It is important to remember that expertise does not provide certainty nor an impartial opinion. Collins and Evans agree that '(o)ne of the paradoxes of expertise is that it might be right to consult it even when the likelihood of its producing correct knowledge is almost zero' (2002: 14).[4] Expert-sources are not 'objective' sources that are above partisan comment. This is demonstrated by the MMR/autism story where Wakefield and pro-MMR scientists were both expert-sources and both had their own viewpoints to publicise.

When researching who is the best person to comment on a story or where is the best place to get background information, the CIN categories can provide journalists with options other than judging a source's availability, prior appearances, articulacy or status. If provided with categories and skills to assess expertise, journalists will be able to answer questions such as:

- What kind of expertise does the source possess?
- Is this expertise related to the story I am writing?
- How can I differentiate between the types of expertise of different sources?
- Does the source have a professional affiliation that might influence them and how their expertise is presented? How independent is the expert-source?
- If the source has no contributory or interactional expertise, am I unfairly balancing it with an expert-source?

Parents' statements should not exclude them from the discussion or, indeed, they should not be excluded from raising questions worthy of systematic research. At the same time, researchers and scientists need to accept that and respond to the fact that personal opinions make complex scientific stories newsworthy. In the case of the MMR/autism story, it is difficult for journalists to 'judge' between parents stating that their child is autistic as a result of the MMR vaccine and scientists telling them there is no scientific evidence that there is a link. Not all knowledge is expert knowledge but journalists must still find a way to represent these different kinds of information. There are signs that in relation to this story, journalists are beginning to see the two types of information as different. On 10 September 2004 new research was published in *The Lancet* confirming the safety of the MMR vaccine. BBC's Radio Five Live's 9:00 phone-in asked the public for their opinions on this latest research. During the hour-long discussion the host challenged a caller who was discussing the stories of parents of autistic children as being powerful statements by saying, 'but how can parents possibly know more than the medical profession?', a question not raised once in the 2002 research sample. Indeed, there are situations where lay people did know more than the so-called experts, as Brian Wynne (1989) astutely recognised with the sheep farmers. The MMR/autism story, however, has become problematic because the knowledge of experts is often abandoned and instead journalists concentrated on the experience and knowledge of a minority of the public who supported the MMR/autism link.

Many factors affect why sources are selected. Sources are selected for their news value, editorial agendas and influences, time pressures or to provide objectivity and balance. Using the definition of expert-sources will not change the reporting of every story, as it is not the only factor when choosing a source. However, particularly in technically complex stories like science, health and risk, considering a source's expertise can help journalists both in selecting the expert-source they quote directly and in selecting those sources used for background information.

CHAPTER EIGHT

Audiences and the MMR/Autism Story

The media coverage of the MMR/autism story had both tangible and subtle effects on parents across the UK. Vaccination levels show exactly how many people have been 'affected' by Wakefield's claims. Prior to Wakefield's 1998 *Lancet* paper, the MMR vaccine uptake had remained at around 90% for a number of years but it fell by more than 10% in the following six years (see Table 1.1 in Chapter 1, page 6). Measuring effect is not as simple as looking only at the vaccination rates: the anxiety caused to parents also needs to be considered as this anxiety can affect future immunisation decisions and attitudes towards expert health advice. The effect of this story is the immediate decline in MMR vaccination levels and also the general decline in trust in the entire vaccination programme. This chapter examines what influenced parents' opinions about the MMR vaccine and their subsequent vaccination decisions. Why did media coverage of the MMR/autism link have such salience among parents? The focus groups and surveys show the public consumed the dominant media frame that the MMR vaccine was unsafe and possibly linked to autism. However, the consumption and reception of this message differed. The audience reaction was not a simple acceptance of this dominant message; the declining vaccination rate shows parents continued to use the MMR vaccine. Parents' vaccination decisions were also informed by information gleaned from sources other than the media.

Stuart Hall's (1980) encoding/decoding theory is used to analyse how mothers responded to and interpreted media coverage. Hall's theory is useful because it argues that meaning does not lie in the text alone, that audiences are active and bring their own opinions, knowledge and experiences when consuming the media. The encoding/decoding theory argues that texts are not endlessly polysemic but that there is a preferred or hegemonic reading, as well as a negotiated position and an oppositional reading. An examination of the different influences and rationales used by parents finds that they fell into each of these positions to varying degrees.

The findings are based on two national surveys and four focus groups. The surveys were carried out in April and October 2002 in 10 locations across the UK.[1] Two focus groups comprised of 30-40 year old middle class mothers, one group of 30 year old working class mothers and one group of teenage mothers. The findings are divided according to parents' vaccination decisions in the following categories:

- "V" (vaccinators) = MMR vaccine given to all children;
- "M" (modifiers) = modified their initial MMR vaccination decision (either single vaccines or no booster or no vaccine to later children);
- "N" (non-vaccinators) = neither MMR nor single vaccines administered to any children.

Each of the focus group participants made a decision about vaccinating a child with the MMR vaccine since Wakefield published his 1998 *Lancet* research. Participants had a total of 40 children, born both before and after the publication of Wakefield's 1998 *Lancet* paper. They chose a range of vaccination strategies, the majority accepting the MMR vaccine, which reflected the national average at the time (see Table 8.1). At the time of the first national survey in April 2002, the MMR uptake was at around 85% (it had reached a high of 92% in the mid-1990s) and dropped slightly by October 2002, when the second survey was completed. By the time of the focus groups in the summer and autumn of 2003, the MMR uptake had fallen below 80%.[2] Previous research finds that when there are periods of intense media coverage, vaccination rates drop (Petts and Niemeyer 2004).

Various health professionals have carried out focus groups with parents to try to understand why MMR vaccination rates have fallen. They found a variety of influences on parents' MMR vaccination decision: past experience of vaccines, confidence and trust in health pro-

Table 8.1 Vaccination status of children of focus group participants

Vaccination	No. Children	Percentage of total
MMR	29	72%
First jab, no booster	7	17%
Single	1	3%
None	3	8%

fessionals, attitudes about choice on immunisation, the views of friends, colleagues and personal attitudes about choice in health care (see, for example, Hobson-West 2003, Rogers 1999, Evans et al. 2001). This research confirms these findings but addresses the role of the media more specifically and its influence and effect in relation to other sources of information.

Influences

The Media

In previous research parents have stated that news media reports are one of their primary sources of information about vaccines and health problems (for an overview see Brown and Walsh-Childers 2002, also Danovaro-Holliday et al. 2002, Singer and Endreny 1987). Health professionals, many of whom are also parents, also regard the mainstream media as a primary source for medical information (Chapman and Lupton 1995, Phillips et al. 1991, Logan 1991). In a poll for *Nursing Times*, 40% of nurses stated the media were the reason for their worries about the MMR vaccine (*Mirror* 14 March 2002). In all focus groups the mothers of young children stated they depended primarily on radio and television for their news; none of the participants regularly read a daily newspaper, stating they did not have the time. The internet and parenting and women's magazines were only identified once.[3] These busy mothers, many of whom had jobs outside the home, claimed they were not heavy news consumers.

For all mothers the media *prompted* them to think about a vaccine they had thought was safe or had given minimum thought to prior to the 1998 publicity.

> Before everything came out in the papers I was quite happy to just go along and have the jabs because it was the normal thing that you did — your children had the MMR and you protected your child.
>
> (M2)

When asked where they got the information they wanted about the MMR vaccine, all focus group participants pointed to the media — 'the news...the media, the radio, the TV it was just saturated (with MMR/autism stories)' (V2). The difference between the mothers was that vaccinators displayed some cynicism of the media coverage and argued the 'media just write what they want, what they think people want to hear about' (V9). They speculated why the MMR/autism story was so attractive to the media, suggesting that the story 'sold papers'.

> Just come up with some flashy headline "MMR is", I don't know, "related to autism" or something we're going to pick it up as parents...It's all about money at the end of the day! (laughter)
>
> (V4)

In another focus group the participants theorised that the media were reporting the story in a particular way; they stated they had heard 'more about the negative side' of the MMR vaccine, with some trying to suggest why this was the case.

> **V2:** It's easier to report the negative sides because it produces more of a reaction.
> **V3:** More interest. (sounds of agreement)
> **V2:** It's more newsworthy, it's produces a reaction.
> **V3:** "MMR is safe" it isn't interesting is it?

These vaccinating mothers viewed the coverage as biased and wanted the media to 'equal them up' (V9), arguing coverage should not just comprise of anti-MMR stories and frames. Other vaccinating parents pointed to the lack of voices heard supporting the vaccine:

> 'What about those people who don't feel their children have been affected by the MMR vaccine? We never hear about that, do we?' (V2).

Even with some awareness of the media's tendency to emphasise the controversial aspects of the story and the anti-MMR side, the parents were open about the media's effect on their thinking, stating, for example, '(The media) made you think about (the MMR/autism link), it was bound to affect your decision' (V5). For vaccinators, the media coverage gave Wakefield's theories validity — if it was in the media, there must be some truth to the story:

Until you hear it through the media you don't know if there might be a problem (voices agree)…But there's always an element of truth whatever you read, there's always an element of truth in it, (it's) not based on complete fabrication is it? It's got to be an element of truth somewhere along the line. So therefore that's what I think you make your decision on.

(V3)

Parents who modified their vaccination decisions or who did not vaccinate at all also openly admitted the media did influence their MMR vaccination decision. Like the vaccinators, they felt coverage granted validity to Wakefield. These parents felt that appearing in the media gives a person or an issue credibility and validity as the media would not deliberately publish untruths. They had faith in the media:

You always feel when it gets into the media there's no smoke without fire and we just looked at the statistics and I personally think there's something going on but it's very difficult isn't it?

(M1)

This parent directly echoes a *Journal of Medical Ethics* editorial written by two scientists who warned that because of the level of media coverage, parents 'have come to the conclusion that there is no smoke without fire' (Clements and Ratzan 2003: 22). If the media simply cover an idea and give it sustained coverage, then the public believes the idea must be authentic and attributes validity to the debate.

Whilst vaccinating, modifying and non-vaccinating parents all referred to the media coverage; there were differences in the level of influence. Modifiers and non-vaccinators were less sceptical of the media and were more disposed to accept the dominant frame, that the MMR vaccine might be dangerous and linked to autism. One teenage mother provided little detail as to why she had chosen not to vaccinate her child; she stated only that she had heard 'it's dangerous' and, upon reflection, stated the media were responsible for her decision not to have the MMR vaccine:

People in the newspapers and all that say it's dangerous and then doctors and all that try and make you have it done.

(N3)

Another mother who had modified her vaccination decision argued that 'with everything being in the news', media coverage had made her 'sit on a wall' as the media had 'put that little bit of doubt in (her) mind' (M2). Several focus group participants commonly stated they did not worry about the MMR vaccine with their first children but 'because there's been more and more and more in the press' (M4) they had changed their minds when considering vaccinating their younger children. Others argued the media's influence was temporary, stating it 'delayed' their decision.

> So if I heard that there was a new outburst on the television I'd think twice, I'd delay it. Delay it again.
>
> (N2)

Clearly the media provided impetus for questioning the safety of the MMR vaccine for all mothers, but non-vaccinating and modifying mothers took media coverage much more seriously and it was more influential in their decisions.

Health Professionals

So if the media caused parents to be concerned about the MMR vaccine, did parents turn elsewhere for further information? For those vaccinators, modifiers and non-vaccinators who sought further information about the MMR vaccine, all turned to their GPs, health visitors, practice nurses and paediatricians. Earlier research in 2001 also found mothers commonly sought advice from health professionals before having their children immunised (Ramsay et al. 2002: 914). In contrast to Evans et al.'s finding that parents felt 'pressure' from health professionals (2001: 907), focus groups participants felt supported by their health professionals—even the non-vaccinators and modifiers—with only one exception. Key to this finding is what parents remembered from these appointments, not scientific information, but the personal opinions of these health professionals.

> **V4:** I remember the health visitor, she was more, "well the government advice is this" and getting out the leaflet (she imitates a leaflet) but then the doctor was like, "well, if it was my child".
> **V5:** Yes, that's the question I always like to ask, what would you do if, it was you?

The type of information that appeals to parents are stories and narratives and 'those…trying to maintain a broader public health perspective need to collect and tell our own stories' (Newman 2003: 1427). Vaccinators were willing to trust the advice from health professionals based on the professionals' personal decisions as well as their expertise.

For vaccinating parents, the main function of health professionals was to alleviate their worries. Vaccinators approached their GPs or health visitors with questions, stating they 'trusted' them to give them 'the right information' (V7).

> I just went and spoke to the nurse in the clinic or the health visitor and said I'm a bit concerned and she just basically gave me a good talking to and said, well you want everyone to have measles, it would be far better if we were all vaccinated. I also spoke to the doctor as well and he just put my mind at rest.
>
> (V4)

Other vaccinators had few questions for health professionals; if the doctor said it was necessary to vaccinate, then they did.

> **TB:** How do you make decisions about his health?
> **V11:** If they say have injections, I have them....
> **V9:** If it weren't safe, they'd take it off wouldn't they? They wouldn't let you go around if they were unsure it was unsafe.

Like the vaccinating parents, modifiers and non-vaccinators also stated they were interested and influenced by the personal choices of their GPs.

> She (GP) had all the medical knowledge but she also had the emotion you know, having children of that age and that whatever she decided I would take her view...like you say doctors and medical people always say oh yes, yes, you know it's alright it's all safe we trust this but you know, she had the emotional side as well.
>
> (M3)

The focus groups revealed that, for the most part, modifiers and non-vaccinators had made the decision not to have the MMR vaccine *without* seeking advice from health professionals. They *assumed* health professionals would recommend the MMR vaccine. As these parents were not making the decision based on 'scientific facts', they were not interested in the arguments from health professionals. The modifiers and non-vaccinators did not entirely reject advice from health professionals but they were less likely to mention them as an influence on their MMR decision. They continued to seek advice from their GPs for other information (other vaccines, illnesses, etc.) but did not do so for the MMR vaccine. Many modifiers and non-vaccinators wanted absolute certainty from health professionals, asking for 'the truth' (N3). One parent, whose older child fully recovered from a severe reaction to the MMR vaccine, wanted a '100% guarantee' that this would not happen with the booster.

Family and Friends

Focus group participants frequently referred to anecdotes from friends or family. The idea that opinion leaders influence the reception of media is long recognised, dating back to Katz and Lazarsfeld's original 1955 research. The two-step flow examines how media messages are mediated through our social relationships and the influence of opinion leaders. Opinion leaders can have significant influences, in the HIV/AIDS story the public frequently turned to 'friends, rather than the mass media, as their source of information' (Miller et al. 1998: 174). The opinions of family and friends can be particularly influential in health stories and emerging issues (Brosius and Weimann 1994, Weimann et al. 2007). In the case of the MMR/autism story, which was an emerging health issue, opinion leaders played an influential role and the mothers of focus group participants were particularly powerful influences.

When vaccinators did respond to their friends' and families' advice they often based this on the friend's or relative's scientific knowledge and not simply because of their relationship.

> (Our family) has somebody who is very high up in the medical profession in this area and I think if he felt that strongly about something like that, knowing we had small children, he would've raised his concerns.
>
> (V8)

When one vaccinating mother discussed the impact of friends with autistic children she referred to views not often heard in the media:

> I know loads of people with autism and I know a lot of people that don't connect it so I've heard other people's stories.
>
> (V9)

Vaccinators were more likely to seek confirmation of their own vaccination decision rather than new information from friends and family. The vaccinators did not always follow what their family members said even though some had a relative who believed there was a link between their child's autism and the MMR vaccine. In one focus group, a vaccinator shared the following story with the group but it provoked no reaction and the group listened and then looked to me for the next question.

(Husband's) cousin's son is severely, severely autistic and he has very chronic bowel problems and they blame that all on the MMR, they said he was fine until then.

(V3)

Whilst previous research found that 'friends and family ranked relatively poorly in terms of trust' (Petts and Niemeyer 2004: 15) when making MMR vaccination decisions, these findings suggest that friends and family, opinion leaders, did influence attitudes towards the MMR vaccine particularly when they possessed scientific expertise.

The most influential opinion leader for vaccinating, modifying and non-vaccinating participants was their mother. One vaccinator discusses how her mother prompted her to worry but her doctor calmed her fears.

I remember there was a double spread in the *Daily Mail* cause my mother kept it for me (laughter)...of a child who suffers from autism, who had the booster and she was like, 'Look, this is the link, look I told you, you know there's a link!' And I'm like, well how many other children in Britain have had the jab and have not got autism? I was trying like, you see, the opposite side, you know, trying to put an argument to her.

(V4)

This was a common experience – it was often mothers of the mothers about to immunise their children who concentrated their minds on the problem. Grandmothers provided recommendations in parenting in general and were 'generalised opinion leaders', who are asked for recommendations in more than one area (Brosius and Weimann 1994: 4). And it was the information the grandmothers had consumed in the media that provoked the focus group participants to worry about the vaccine. Considering the significant impact of grandmothers' practice of sending articles to their adult children, perhaps researchers examining the opinions of vaccinating parents should ask not only what they read, but also what their mother reads!

Conversely, family and friends had little impact for modifiers and non-vaccinators. Few of these parents referred to conversations with friends and family and did not discuss that they had spoken to them when making their MMR decision. In addition to friends and family having a less significant influence for non-vaccinators and modifiers, the *type* of information they looked for from friends and family differed from those who vaccinated with the MMR vaccine. The vaccinators referred to scientific evidence from friends and family, whereas the non-vaccinators and modifiers wanted personal information, specifically whether they had vaccinated their children with the MMR vaccine. Here a modifying mother refers to a friend, a medical doctor, who influenced her decision and it is the decision, not the scientific evidence or reasons, that interested her:

> In the end, I spoke to very good friend of mine who's a GP with a child the same age as (her son) and one slightly younger and I said, you know, what are you doing, what do you think? And that was, she was my conscience.
>
> (M3)

Focus group discussions revealed that those who declared early in the discussions not to have spoken to anyone else or claimed not to have been worried about the MMR vaccine eventually revealed they had turned to social networks to discuss the issue, usually their partner, family, friends or a health professional.

Their Own Science Knowledge

Few focus group participants stated they based their decision only on their own knowledge or experiences. The few who claimed they spoke to no one or referred to no other materials all contradicted themselves later in the discussion. Much has been written about the 'informed patient' making decisions about their health but this discourse 'assumes that individuals want to take more and more responsibility for their own health' (Henwood et al. 2004: 81). The focus groups established that parents infrequently sought information beyond visiting their GP, thus challenging the idea that patients want to take more responsibility about their own health care.

Both the national survey results and focus group findings demonstrate that the level of science education had a modest influence on their MMR vaccine decision. Table 8.2 shows those with A-Level science education or above were more likely to choose the MMR vaccine.

Attitudes to and knowledge about the MMR vaccine were affected by levels of science education. Many focus group participants were aware of basic information, for instance, the proposed link with autism, but they were unaware of more detailed scientific information. Survey respondents with an A Level or higher were more likely to know that the controversy involved a proposed link between the vaccine and autism rather than any other disorder and that the majority of evidence suggested no link with the MMR vaccine (see Figure 8.1).

Table 8.2 If you were making a decision on whether to vaccinate a child against measles, mumps and rubella, what would you choose?[4]

	A level or higher	GCSE/O Level	None
MMR vaccine	56%	53%	43%
3 Separate injections	32%	28%	31%
No vaccination	1%	4%	6%
Don't know	11%	15%	20%

In the focus groups all those with A-Level or higher science education opted for the MMR vaccine and did not question the science given to them by health professionals. Those who had a science background (V5, V7, V1) often turned to that background when justifying their decision and also discussed their education when trying to show others what information was available.

> **V1:** But babies' immune systems work different to adults' immune system, that's the whole point. That's why you give babies, that's why you give (vaccines) when they're young.
> **V3:** But it's different for you, because you know, you're a medical person.
> **V1:** Yes, you're right.
> **V3:** You've got a totally medical background and you know everything!
> **V1:** I don't know everything!
> **V3:** You do! (laughter)

Focus group participants with scientific backgrounds still spoke to their health professionals and were more likely to trust this information.

> I guess I've got a bit of a different background to everybody else because I've got a science background I kind of understand what a clinical trial is and that sort of thing. So I've got a bit more background understanding than the average person anyway.
>
> (V5)

Very few focus group participants blamed themselves or their lack of scientific knowledge for their erroneous understandings of the MMR/autism link; instead they blamed the media. Upon being told that Wakefield's research was based on 12 children and not a larger sample, a mother reacted with anger and surprise:

> **M3:** If that is true I'm disgusted…
> **TB:** Why are you disgusted? Who are you disgusted with?

M3: (pause) The media I suppose, I don't know. I think well yes, if he was at a press conference and that was reported well it's come from no where else.

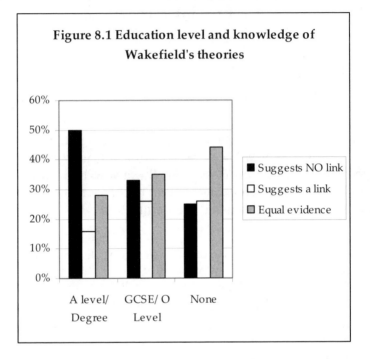

Figure 8.1 Education level and knowledge of Wakefield's theories

And later in this focus group one mother complains that 'There should've been a headline this was based on twelve cases but there wasn't was there?' (M4). As the media analysis showed, the media generally failed to discuss the details of Wakefield's research. One focus group participant with science education and who knew the research very well[5] was clear that the media coverage was misleading and argued that it had led to people misunderstanding the amount of evidence.

> **V5:** I think it's kinda been forgotten that only one research group came up with this hypothesis and everybody else in the world didn't agree with him, so I think it's one group or one man against everybody else.
> **TB:** What do you think?
> **M2:** Um. I'm gonna have to pass on that one cause I've not heard of this (Wakefield) chap.
> **V5:** There we are then, that proves my point!

This issue of the public's lack of knowledge of the evidence supporting Wakefield's claim also raises another significant issue. The second survey in October 2002 included a question about maverick scientists asking if the media should report their research findings (which often challenge the status quo) or wait until this research is confirmed by further research (see Figure 8.2). The survey results showed a mixed reaction with half wanting the media to wait until further research confirms the controversial findings. But the focus groups showed that the public *did not think Wakefield's views were 'maverick' views*, and they did not know that Wakefield had so little evidence or support from the scientific community. That scientists and researchers labelled Wakefield as a maverick did not transmit to many members of the audience, who instead saw media coverage as evidence that his views were credible.

The findings from the focus groups relate in interesting ways to current debates in the field of public understanding of science. The traditional public understanding of science theory assumes that the more knowledge the public possesses the more likely they are to support scientific endeavours. Later research found the contrary, that more information can lead to increased *concern* about science and technology and therefore a *decline* in support (see, for instance, Frewer and Shepherd 1994, Evans and Durant 1995, INRA Europe 2000). However, in this study, both the focus groups and national surveys show that those with higher levels of science education were more likely to select the MMR vaccine. Increased knowledge led to an increase, not a decline, in support of specific medical interventions. Therefore, one should not assume that more knowledge inevitably leads to more scepticism.

Journalists' Views of Their Role and Their Audience

Journalists had mixed opinions about their influence over the audience; some admitted the audience might make decisions based on their stories whilst others stated they provided 'information' but were not 'educating' audiences. When challenged, journalists were unable to explain the difference between providing 'information' and 'educating' the audience. For those who did accept they were educating their audience, they felt this pressure when reporting.

> Every time you write you're thinking some poor bugger's just had their lung cancer diagnosed or just about to go to their GP...I'm really very careful and low key about this particular story because of the vaccination problem... In

terms of being right, in terms of getting your facts right. We need to be extremely responsible about this.

(Health editor)

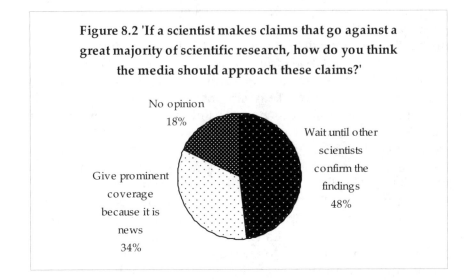

Figure 8.2 'If a scientist makes claims that go against a great majority of scientific research, how do you think the media should approach these claims?'

But not all journalists agreed that they had such a powerful influence on their audience. One journalist felt she had a responsibility to be pro-MMR but was resolute that she had no way of knowing if her stories had any 'effect'.

> **TB:** In terms of being a health correspondent, do you feel that people are making decisions based on what you write, are you educating the public?
> **Journalist:** I don't know, I can't tell you, you'd have to do an opinion poll...I simply do my job to the best of my ability by telling people what I think is an accurate representation of the way things are, or at the very least, showing the different views so that they can decide for themselves...I don't know whether people are influenced—I just don't—it's impossible to say as a journalist actually.
>
> (Health editor)

When asked to imagine their audience, journalists turned to professional practices to describe the level they pitch their stories at.

> You know you're always writing for your mom and your sister and your auntie aren't you—who don't have a medical background. So I must neither patronise my reader by making it over-simple or making it too complicated...They want their own opinions confirmed.
>
> (Health editor)

Individual journalists stated they did not have the time to examine any impact from their stories. Instead, they regarded their duty to relay information and to mediate information between sources and audiences. Journalists were more concerned about performing these tasks well than any potential effects their stories might have on their audiences.

Rationales

The following section examines the rationales used by parents to defend their MMR vaccination decision. Three main rationales are discussed: the fear of autism, the fear of measles, mumps and rubella and concepts of trust and risk. Also included is a short analysis of two secondary rationales: herd immunity and overloading immune systems.

Fear of Autism

All focus group participants repeatedly referred to their fear of autism when discussing their MMR vaccination decision. Their fear of autism was discussed more frequently than their fear of measles, mumps and rubella and discussions of autism elicited more animated responses. When asked what they remembered about the coverage, 'autism' was the immediate response from focus group participants.

> There were *rumours about autism*...That he might develop autism after the MMR.
>
> (V10)

The national surveys asked the public which medical disorder was linked to the MMR vaccine. Two-thirds of respondents correctly identified 'autism' (see Table 8.3) and very few answered the question incorrectly. This suggests a high awareness of the link (older and younger respondents were more likely to answer 'don't know' to this question as they are less likely to have direct relationships with young children at vaccination age).

Table 8.3 Some recent research has suggested there might be a link between the MMR vaccine and which medical disorder?

	April (n=1035)	October (n=1037)
Autism	67%	66%
Down's Syndrome	8%	7%
Blindness	3%	4%
Dyslexia	2%	2%
Don't know	21%	22%

Autism has become part of the standard discourse when discussing the MMR vaccine, even for vaccinators. The simple repetition of the claim that there might be a link to autism planted an image in the audiences' minds. The quantity of coverage can have just as a can have just as a significant effect as semantic content: 'the public takes seriously any suggestion that technology may be risky, particularly if the suggestion is repeated often enough' (Mazur 1981: 114). When one mother states she thinks measles, mumps and rubella are 'serious' diseases (V10) a non-vaccinating mother immediately responds, 'she might get autism', as if the choice is between measles, mumps and rubella or autism. Another vaccinating mother also refers to the advice given to her by her GP and her mother but then states the most significant issue for her:

> The doctor said, 'well we remember measles as children ourselves and it's an awful thing'. And my mother said the same thing as well — but no, for me the biggest thing was the autism.
>
> (V4)

If the focus groups were *concerned* about autism, very few had knowledge of autism and few were aware that the causes of autism remain unknown.

> **V2:** What about going back to autism, yeah, I mean they're talking about autism being, there has to be a reason and sometimes there isn't?
> **M1:** As far as autism itself, I'm not an expert in it or anything like that but autism is a new-ish thing isn't it? I can't ever remember.
> **V2:** I think people are more, more aware and more knowledgeable about diagnosing, they're more knowledgeable about labelling the certain condition aren't they?

They questioned each other and asked me for information on autism but it was clear from the focus groups that the information they possessed regarding autism came primarily from the media and, secondly, from friends' and family's experiences.[6]

In addition to the perceived risk of having an autistic child was the fear that if their child developed autism, they would feel responsible because they had sanctioned the vaccination. This issue was raised by Dr. Mike Fitzpatrick, father of an autistic child and a GP. Fitzpatrick accused Wakefield of making parents of autistic children, who already feel tired and unsupported, believe they are responsible for their child's disorder. The idea that they could not 'forgive themselves', that they might be to blame for their child's autism, was prevalent among all focus group participants and one mother lamented how difficult the decision was, referring to the guilt she felt when trying to make the decision.

> But I think that is a big issue especially with what's happening you know, with MMR. You know if it was linked to autism, how could you ever forgive yourself? ('Mmms' from others) …I think that is a huge, huge issue for me. That was the biggest issue.
>
> (M3)

The images of autistic children, more so their exhausted and frustrated parents, were prominent images when parents discussed the MMR vaccine. It was much more than simply the effect of the disease on the child that terrified focus group participants; it was the impact autism would have on their own lives and their families' lives. In one group the fear of autism dominated the discussion and one mother summed up her view:

> I remember my sister saying to me years ago and she's worked with autistic young people for all of her life, she was saying I would be devastated if I had an autistic child because the social connection isn't there.
>
> (V6)

As Miller et al. argue, 'it is not just language, silences, narrative structures and cultural baggage that are important; visual images are also crucial' (1998: 178). For modifiers and non-vaccinators, the media images of autistic children also had a significant impact, with one stating that parents of autistic children who blamed the MMR vaccine 'influenced my thinking' (M4) and another stated:

> You know people who's children have been affected and suspect that it was from the vaccine… I think for me that's what the pivotal thing is, the issue.
>
> (M3)

As well as referring to media coverage of these tired parents of autistic children, participants also held a collective memory of autistic children which was acquired from their own social networks and experiences. The images of children damaged by measles, mumps and rubella did not figure for parents when they made the MMR vaccine decision: instead the dominant image was of autistic children. Whether or not the participants believed the claims of parents of autistic children that the MMR vaccine was responsible, they were nonetheless exceptionally affected by these emotional statements, stating it influenced their thinking.

> The parents who have autistic children...that was more shocking, more, it had a bigger impact on me because you could see what may happen. Your child is normal, you want them to stay as they are, you don't want them to develop autism, you know your life is being turned upside down.
>
> (V4)

Not once did focus group participants refer to children with measles, mumps or rubella or the impact these diseases would have on the lives of parents. Media coverage provided powerful images of autism, leaving a lasting impression on the focus group participants. This fear caused one non-vaccinator to be emphatic that *their* child would not be *forced* into a position which might result in autism.

> Ok, it hasn't been proven (link between MMR and autism) but equally you're still battling against people like me who are not going to give their child MMR. Whatever! No way! It's not going to happen!...The bottom line is that I'm not prepared to give my child MMR in case he gets autism.
>
> (N1)

Some vaccinators, even after reassurance from medical professionals, continued to believe there might be a link between MMR and autism but chose the MMR vaccine instead because, as outlined below, they believed the dangers of the diseases were greater or trusted advice from health professionals.

For modifiers and non-vaccinators, fear of autism superseded any fear of measles, mumps or rubella, and this, combined with their distrust of science and government, resulted in their choice to vaccinate with single vaccines or not to vaccinate at all. The 'choice' to have single vaccines or the triple MMR jab was attractive to parents because audiences respond differently to risks they choose themselves over those which they believe they have some degree of control over (Klaidman 1990: 126).

Detailed Rationales 1: Overloading the Immune System

Whilst few focus group participants referred to Wakefield's theories in any detail, one of Wakefield's scientific arguments did resonate with focus group participants: that a child's immune system could be 'overwhelmed' by giving three vaccines at one time. Wakefield's assertions were not supported by any medical evidence; instead this was a hypothesis he promoted in the media after publishing the 1998 *Lancet* paper.[7] A number of focus group participants raised this part of Wakefield's hypothesis, using it to legitimise their vaccination choice. They measured the health of their child's immune system themselves by physically looking at their children or remembering their previous illnesses. Pro-vaccination parents were generally less concerned about this issue but a small number of vaccinators did raise this issue. One parent describes when she decided it was 'safe' to vaccinate her children—after observing her child's health.

> I made sure that they were exceptionally healthy at the time of having any vaccinations carried out. If they had the slightest temperature or you know anything, even just practically just looked a bit wiped out for the day, I wouldn't take them. I made sure they were a 100% when they went in and I just hoped for the best I think.
>
> (V8)

The idea of the health of a child's immune system was part of the standard discourse for non-vaccinators or modifiers.

> My husband was really set against a really young baby having MMR, because (he) wanted their immune system to be stronger.
>
> (N2)

Why were the participants so ready to accept the idea that the immune system might be overwhelmed by the triple vaccine? Was it simply a lack of understanding of how the immune system works? Overloading the immune system only occurred in 1% of stories in the research period, so where did parents get this information from? Lupton identifies general increasing media coverage of the immune system in Western culture (2003: 68). This issue might also be evidence that parents obtained information from sources other than the media. In addition, the idea that the immune system could be overwhelmed was perhaps more understandable for focus group participants who believed they could measure their child's immune system simply by looking at them. The idea of assessing the strength or weakness of a child seemed to find resonance with focus group participants and middle class parents in particular.

Fear of Measles, Mumps and Rubella

When focus group participants considered the risks from the MMR vaccine versus the risks from the three diseases the vaccine protects from, what was clear was that they lacked information about measles, mumps and rubella. Petts and Niemeyer similarly found that when they showed DoH videos about the MMR vaccine to their focus group participants, the 'most commonly cited pieces of "new" learning were in relation to the side effects of the three diseases' (2004: 16). Part of the reason for this was the success of the vaccination programme itself, as few parents had recent memories of measles, mumps or rubella. One of the DoH's key messages was the dangers of these three diseases; however, the communication of this message appears to have failed, as most parents in the focus groups lacked knowledge of these diseases and referred to them as mild or were ignorant of the potential seriousness of the diseases. One group possessed little knowledge of the dangers of the diseases and asked me directly 'what happens if you get mumps or rubella?'

Even if many focus group participants did not know the repercussions of the diseases, for vaccinators, the idea that children needed protection from diseases was a constant theme. In the following exchange, V1, a medical doctor, questions her friends' knowledge of the dangers of mumps. Prior to this, mumps was being discussed as a *mild* disease.

> **V1:** I mean, do you know why they give mumps vaccines?
> (extended pause)
> **V3:** Why they give what?
> **TB:** Do you know the danger of mumps?
> **N2:** I know that if a boy has mumps (it) might cause him to be sterile.
> **V1:** Yes, sterile.
> **N1:** But that's very unusual in adult males, I thought it was more to do with the danger of encephalitis than with.
> **V1:** (interrupts) It is, but it's quite a large proportion of men who become sterile after the mumps. When I used to do the infertility clinic a large proportion of those coming had had mumps when they were kids.
> **V3:** Really?

The only disease discussed in detail in focus groups was measles. Rubella and mumps were rarely mentioned, perhaps reflecting the lack of media coverage of these two diseases. When remembering the effects of measles, the focus group participants discussed personal stories and told stories about measles.

> I'm sure actually it was the nurse in the clinic who pointed this out to me and she remembers when measles was around when she was a youngster and my mother pointed that out as well. It was far better to have the kids all vaccinated rather to them have measles and mumps back because it's just awful.
>
> (V4)

> A very good friend of mine nearly died of measles when she was a baby when she was 2 months old so that was a deciding factor with me. (Friend), that was the deciding factor.
>
> (V6)

When focus group participants did discuss their own experiences or memories of the diseases, they had few to share because of the success of the vaccination programmes which have made these diseases rare in the UK. One of the repercussions of a successful vaccination policy is that people forget the dangers of the diseases. As such, Clements and Ratzan argue that parents 'are reverting to the belief that it is safer to have the disease than have their children vaccinated' and that the diseases are not 'serious' (2003: 22).

Even though many had little detailed information about the dangers or risks of measles, mumps and rubella, the vaccinators nonetheless feared their children catching one of the diseases and this very much influenced their decision to vaccinate. One mother discussed her own experiences of measles and whooping cough and declared, 'I think I would rather have an autistic child than a dead child. Sorry for being so blunt (laughs)' (V8). One teenage mother challenged another about forgetting the dangers of the diseases:

> V9: But surely you'd rather have a kid with autism than not have a kid at all?
> N3: Well, what if she turns out autistic?
> V9: What if she gets measles, mumps or rubella?

The modifiers and non-vaccinators had different opinions of the diseases than the vaccinators. Modifiers and non-vaccinators were either unaware of the seriousness of the diseases or believed they were mild and rare. In contrast to the mother above, another asked, 'She can't die from the diseases can she?' (N3). One mother argued it was a 'less important' vaccination and defended her view:

> While they're all dangerous, it's difficult to see them (measles, mumps and rubella) as that dangerous when we all had it and we're all fine. I don't know, but that was another reason, maybe that was easier not to have that than not to have others.
>
> (M4)

Particularly for modifiers and non-vaccinators, basing their MMR decision on their own personal experience of measles was common: the 'I survived it, why won't my children?' attitude was a frequent refrain.

The dangers of the diseases was a rationale used by focus group participants to justify both their decision to vaccinate or not vaccinate. Focus group participants did not directly weigh up the risks of measles versus the risk of autism, but it was more a matter of what they feared more—measles, mumps and rubella or autism.

Detailed Rationales 2: Herd Immunity

Research has consistently found that the herd immunity argument is an ineffective way of convincing parents to vaccinate their children (e.g., Rogers and Pilgrim 1995, Hobson-West 2003). During the interview with the DoH representative, he stated that the DoH's research showed that parents were not concerned with the benefits immunisation brought to wider society and only considered their own situation when making vaccination decisions. However, some focus group participants stated they were influenced by the herd immunity argument. One parent described how her doctor and health visitor tried to convince her:

> Their argument was mainly based on it's better to have the immunisation so measles doesn't come back.
>
> (V4)

Others understood why herd immunity was a desirable goal:

> 'I think you have a responsibility to vaccinate your child because there are weaker children that need to be protected'.
>
> (V6)

Modifiers and non-vaccinators, on the whole, did not discuss herd immunity and were only concerned for their own children. This was clearly illustrated when one group was told that the child of one of the participants suffered from leukaemia and was therefore more susceptible to the three diseases. One non-vaccinating parent showed some concern for this child but stated her ultimate concern was for the health of her own child.

> **V1:** I suppose I have a different view because my child is immuno-suppressed so if (son) got measles that would be it...At the moment we're ok because there's not a measles epidemic or mumps so if you don't immunise your child the chances of him actually getting it are... But in a few years time, that's going to be really difficult because the chances of him getting measles, mumps and rubella are going to be very real because the vaccination rate is going to have dropped so much so there really will be a difficult decision. Now you can just fight by saying there's no measles around here, chances of getting it are virtually nil...
>
> **N1:** The bottom line is though and you've made me think about having single vaccines. What you've just said is, made me think, oh shit. The bottom line is the choice is not easily there for me to have and that is the bottom line for me — is that the choice for single vaccine should be there.

The DoH's decision not to use herd immunity as a key message seems to be supported by the focus group data, as it would appear that this argument would not alter the decision of non-vaccinating parents. However, for those who supported the MMR, the herd immunity argument validated their choice and made them feel like they were making their communities safer for all.

Trust

In focus groups, participants described their concerns, anger and frustration with institutions and politicians and their dilemma about who to trust for information about the MMR vaccine. Public opinion of doctors and scientists remains fairly positive as numerous public polls identify a 'GP' or 'doctor' as the most trustworthy profession in society and other polls point to the faith the public has in science (e.g., INRA Europe 2000, Hargreaves et al. 2003). The national surveys attempted to measure attitudes towards science and found, as many other polls have found, that the public, on the whole, trusts science and believes it is acting in the collective interests of society (see Table 8.4).

Research argues that the reason why there is declining trust in science is because of previous issues such as GM foods, foot-and-mouth, BSE, mobile phones, etc. (Clements and Ratzan 2003: 22, Evans et al. 2001). In light of this, the national survey asked an open-ended question about reasons for this supposed declining trust in science. Just over half the public stated that trust in science had decreased and named a variety of reasons for this decline (see Figure 8.3). Many survey respondents, almost half, stated that nothing had decreased their trust in science. Few focus group participants mentioned any of these issues in the focus groups; BSE was only briefly mentioned in two focus groups.

Table 8.4 Which of the following do you think is the main aim of most scientific research?

	October
To improve human life	70%
To satisfy the curiosity of scientists	11%
To benefit business	11%
Don't know	8%

In any discussions of the public and trust, researchers need to consider the respondents' answers with caution. As Frewer and Shepherd argue, 'stated trust in hypothetical information sources does not necessarily correspond with trust in the same sources in an actual or simulated context' (1994: 397). In focus groups, concepts of trust were difficult to understand and disentangle. Vaccinating parents stated they simply trusted their health care professionals' advice because they had the knowledge and expertise.

> I trusted my health visitor to give me the right information.
>
> (V7)

In one focus group, parents discussed their trust in television doctors, but why they were trustworthy was difficult to unravel. When asked who they might trust to talk to them about the MMR vaccine, they answered:

> **V4:** Dr Hilary Jones (laughter)
> **TB:** Carter from ER? (laughter)
> **V5:** Yeah, that would be nice!
> **M2:** Somebody who knows.
> **TB:** Who is that? Tell me who is somebody who knows?...
> **V4:** I'm thinking Dr. Chris Steele (laughs) I always trust whatever he says, do you know Dr. Chris Steele he used to be on 'This Morning' and I don't know if he still is...
> **M2:** I don't trust any of the doctors on television...
> **V5:** He looks trustworthy though doesn't he?

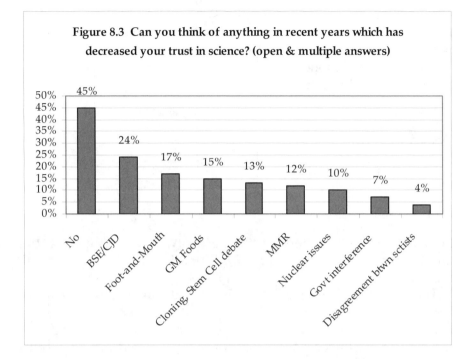

Figure 8.3 Can you think of anything in recent years which has decreased your trust in science? (open & multiple answers)

'Looking' trustworthy was enough for some parents, or even just appearing on a popular morning magazine programme. Focus group participants argued they trusted scientists to take the public's best interests to heart and depended on scientists to be open about potential dangers of the MMR vaccine. One parent trusted the British Medical Association to inform the public.

> (The BMA and) all these people getting paid massive amounts of money to investigate such scares and I would hope they would highlight any problems with these vaccinations. I think you have to trust somebody like that at the end of the day because that's what they're paid to find out. And inform us via GPs and then they can inform the people who read *The Sun*, that *The Sun* is, in fact, incorrect.
>
> (V8)

In contrast to the vaccinators, parents who had modified their vaccination decision or decided not to vaccinate stated they had little trust in government and scientific advice. Modifiers and non-vaccinators were keen to state they were *willing* to trust but unsure *who* to trust.

> I tend to rely more on what people tell me because they're in the profession and they should know. I'm quite trusting like that.
>
> (M2)

For some modifiers, even when they stated they did trust their GPs, they still decided not to vaccinate with the MMR vaccine. In the following example, M4 vaccinated her first two children with the MMR vaccine, and even though she finds her GP 'nice' and 'trusted him', she nonetheless chose single vaccines for her third child.

> **M4:** He (GP) reassured that it was safe and you should have it.
> **V6:** It's what they (GP) all say.
> **M4:** Yes and you sort of know that's what they're gonna say
> but he was very nice and I trusted him.
> **V8:** I think they're more informed.
> **M4:** Exactly.
> **V8:** Than us.
> **M4:** I'm quite trusting.

The above example underlines the difficulty of assessing trust; this parent states that she trusts her GP but not their advice on the MMR vaccine.

The most significant reason for the lack of trust in science was the focus group participants' view of apparent government interference in science. If parents were unsure who to trust, they were clear who they did not trust—the government or any perceived interference by them. Parents from all four groups blamed a general distrust of authorities and government interference as a reason why they were confused as to who to trust on this issue.

> I think there's a distrust of authorities saying it's alright. I think that's my partner's problem, is that anyone saying anything different, he's just, has got a natural distrust of the official line. He's the same about all health scares, believes the scare and doesn't believe the reassurances and I think probably a lot of people are like that.
>
> (M4)

To a large extent, parents' cynicism of the government on this issue can be attributed to Tony Blair's refusal to state whether or not he had vaccinated his youngest child. This issue resonated with the audience in focus groups and in the surveys. A question about Blair's position received the highest number of correct answers in both of the surveys, with 66% of respondents in April correctly answering that 'The Prime Minister has stated that this is a private matter' which rose to 70% in October (see Table 8.5).

Table 8.5 Which of the following statements is true?

	April (n=1035)	October (n=1037)
The PM's son, Leo Blair, has had the MMR vaccine	23%	17%
The PM's son, Leo Blair, has NOT had the MMR vaccine	8%	11%
The PM has stated that this is a private matter	66%	70%

Three of the four focus groups brought up Tony Blair without prompting. Focus group participants were not only knowledgable about Leo's vaccination status but most, particularly the modifiers and non-vaccinators, were frustrated and angry that Blair did not discuss his decision.

> **M4:** Which makes me think of the Blair issue. I think that put a lot of big questions in people's minds when they wouldn't come out and say whether their child had been vaccinated or not. It had (a) huge influence even though it was perfectly within their rights not to say whether they had it or not cause it's nothing to do with anyone…I do think that they influenced people, the fact that they wouldn't come out and say they're going to have the MMR…
> **V6:** And it was a perfect opportunity for him really to lead on that. Surprisingly they didn't, so they obviously, they didn't give it to him did they? Possibly. Do you know?
> **V7:** I'm gobsmacked that he didn't come out and say that they'd had it.

Focus group participants argued that knowing Blair's decision would have influenced their own, as they believed he had access to information they did not.

> **M1:** I think if Tony Blair had said, look I've had it done, people would think, I would think, he must have access to the best information. (Yeah from others), he would've had the biggest range of information.
> **V3:** And people running around looking into it.
> **M1:** Top advisors, yeah, exactly. That he would've really done his homework because he's got access to everything.

If Leo Blair had been given the MMR vaccine, the focus group findings suggest that the Prime Minister's refusal to disclose this information, whilst understandable on a personal level, was, in public health terms, (at least in the short term) a mistake. It kept open the possibility that the Prime Minister had reviewed the evidence and decided *against* the MMR jab, which can only have added to people's fears.[8]

Influence of Gender

Gender had a significant impact on how the MMR/autism story was consumed. In the focus groups, both mothers and fathers were invited to participate; however, only mothers agreed to do so. One father sat in on the teenage mothers' focus group but said nothing, even when asked directly. During two focus groups held in the homes of participants, fathers were at home but declined to participate. Some mothers referred to conversations with their partners, but more typically they remarked that they made vaccination and health decisions about their children on their own.

> I was with (son's) dad at the time and well, basically, explained to him my worries and he was like, well, you decide and that was it. (laughter) Thanks for that!
>
> (V4)

> Well I made the choice on my own. I discussed this with my husband last week and asked whether I mentioned it to him and he said no I didn't and I just went ahead and did it, which is what I normally do.
>
> (V8)

The national surveys revealed that a relatively equal number of women and men would choose the MMR vaccine, that is, 51% of women and 49% of men. However, the focus groups revealed that mothers (and their mothers) were the key decision makers for the MMR vaccine. These findings suggest that more attention might need to be paid to exploring who are the key decision makers about vaccination and the information provided to (and by) women. For instance, knowing that mothers were more influential in making vaccination decisions makes certain statistics much more revealing. Table 8.6 reveals how many more women than men knew that recent research claimed a linked between the MMR vaccine and autism.

Table 8.6 Some recent research has suggested there might be a link between the MMR vaccine and which medical disorder?

	Female	Male
Autism	75%	57%
Don't Know	16%	27%
Down's Syndrome	5%	9%
Blindness	3%	4%
Dyslexia	1%	3%

Media Effects?

The focus groups and surveys reveal the difference between the 'interpretation of' and 'reaction to' the MMR/autism story (Kitzinger 1998). If the majority of the audience was aware of the MMR/autism controversy, why did only parts of the audience change their vaccination decisions? What made some parents choose single vaccines or no MMR vaccination whilst the majority continued to choose the MMR vaccine?

One factor provided the modifiers and non-vaccinators with their reason for rejecting the MMR vaccine: the fear of autism. For vaccinating parents, fear of the three diseases, trust in the safety of the MMR vaccine and trust in health professionals were their main rationales. Parents did not weigh up the risks of autism versus the risks of measles, mumps or rubella because they did not know the dangers of the diseases.

If audience responses could be reduced to three main groups—vaccinators, modifiers and non-vaccinators—does this suggest there were limits to the text's polysemous nature? As Condit (1989) argues, there are limits to an audience's ability to shape their own readings of a text. The main reason why the audience was limited in its understanding of the MMR/autism story was that the work required to decode the media coverage was onerous, especially for busy mothers. Access to material in medical journals that might form an oppositional or negotiated code were difficult for the general public to access and understand. That the majority of the audience continued to vaccinate does not advocate that audience activity necessarily diminishes media influence because the audience *did* worry and anxiety increased. As Lewis argues, media influence is not tempered; instead media influence is 'more complex and diffuse' (2001: 85).

Hall's encoding/decoding theory helps us to understand the differing impact of the media on vaccinators, modifiers and non-vaccinators. Hall's theory rejects textual determinism and argues 'decodings do not follow inevitably from encodings' (1980: 136). In the MMR/autism story, the audience's multiple responses demonstrated that the way the story was decoded did not automatically follow how the story was encoded. The analysis of the media coverage showed that the preferred meaning of the story was that the MMR vaccine might be unsafe and linked to autism. The preferred reading accepted that the MMR vaccine might be unsafe because the science evidence was believable and the sources stating the vaccine was safe could not be trusted. Those who accepted the preferred reading were the non-vaccinating parents who rejected the triple vaccine and either chose single vaccines or no vaccination. In general, modifiers and non-vaccinators spoke to fewer friends and family and some did not discuss their concerns with their health professionals. Instead, their overwhelming fear of autism and confusion over who to trust were more salient influences.

The majority of parents continued to vaccinate their children with the MMR vaccine, and the media had an inconsistent influence on them. These parents worried about the MMR vaccine's safety, but instead of straight acceptance of this message, they based their decisions on other information or remembered past experiences of the vaccine: they *negotiated* the preferred meaning in the media. This was the most common experience of mothers in focus groups. When one mother states, 'I'd read it, I'd watch it whatever but I'd still make my own decision based on my own thoughts' (V5), she does not openly state the extent of the media influence but implicitly acknowledges that it played a part in her decision-making process. Some parents admitted they were easily swayed by information in the media. Towards the end of their focus group, these middle class, university-educated parents admitted:

> **V2:** But sometimes it's the last thing that you hear you know and I'm as guilty as much as everyone else...But if you hear a compelling argument for and you think oh god, I really agree with what they say and you hear an equally compelling argument against, sometimes it's the last argument you hear. Cause you identify with both.
> **V3:** And you therefore tend to quote it if you're talking about it.
> **V2:** So is it if you hear more against are you more likely to identify with that argument?...

V1: I can't think of an example but if somebody comes on to the telly about something and I think yeah that's absolutely true!
V3: Well I'm a bit like that...I think we all tend to go oh yeah (head on one side) and then oh yeah. (head on other side)

Parents who negotiated the dominant framework of the media coverage accepted the idea that the MMR vaccine might be unsafe, but then spoke to health professionals, family and friends in order to help them make their decision. They brought to their reception of the MMR/autism story their prior opinions of the MMR vaccine, knowledge and their relationships with their family, friends, GP or midwife. They used these experiences, knowledge and relationships when negotiating information from the media. New information is often understood in ways that support an individual's pre-existing views (Thomas 1997: 171). One participant suggested that people are more likely to maintain their attitude based on information they already possess.

> The position you start at, isn't that going to be the position you end at? If you have a start position that is heavily weighted by the pro-argument then any arguments against is going to have less influence than if you started at the other end of the scale.
>
> (V2)

A much smaller group of parents rejected the dominant frame outright. The oppositional code was to believe the MMR vaccine was safe, thus rejecting the dominant media frame that it might be linked to autism. For parents who challenged this media frame, the dangers of measles, mumps and rubella was more significant than any link to autism and they were more likely to trust information from science and government. Fewer parents were in this group, but there were some who stated:

> The (media coverage) didn't affect me, cause I'd already made my decision.
>
> (V8)

Large parts of the audience displayed some resistance to the dominant media frame and sought reassurance from GPs, friends and family. The MMR vaccination rate did drop and parents' level of concern increased, but on the whole, the vaccination rate showed that the majority of parents continued to choose the MMR vaccine. But the focus groups also revealed that the dominant ideology of undermining science persisted; even if the audience did oppose the preferred meaning of the text, resistance did not result in the rejection of the preferred reading. When the audience displayed scepticism of science and government sources, this was often because of the confusion that arose as a result of trying to understand the disagreement between these sources.

In the MMR/autism story, agenda-setting theory applies in particular to journalists, whose experience of reporting previous science controversies now shapes how they report current science stories. In the case of the MMR vaccine, the agenda-setting effect of the media on parents was more complex. In classic agenda-setting theory, Cohen (1963) argued that the media do not tell people what to think, but what to think about. Since Cohen's original statements about media influence, agenda-setting theory has evolved and research shows the media can have a profound influence on audiences and that 'the media are instrumental in providing information and that 'one's store of information shapes one's opinions' (McCombs, Danielian and Wanta 1995: 295 in Lewis 2001). By simply telling parents to 'think about' the fact that the MMR vaccine might be 'unsafe' led to parents 'thinking' this vaccine was dangerous. When the media introduce new ideas or discussions—for example, that the MMR vaccine might cause autism—the media become important sources of information, as the media make the public '*think the unthinkable*' (Kitzinger 2004). In the case of the MMR/autism story, media coverage introduced parents to the idea that the triple vaccine might be unsafe. One vaccinating parent admits she worried because of the media coverage.

> If I were doing it now, I think because I have seen lots of headlines and my understanding of the media is very minimal cause I distrust it…but I think because there are more headlines around I think I would ask more questions at this point than I did back then.
>
> (V7)

That the media acted as a catalyst, asking the public to 'think the unthinkable' was evident in all four focus groups.

> I think if it weren't all in the media and all that then I'd've had it done.
>
> (N3)

Prior to the 1998 *Lancet* publication the MMR vaccine rarely appeared in the media. Parents trusted the vaccine and uptake was high. When the MMR vaccine received significant media coverage after the *Lancet* article, parents started to worry about a vaccine they had previously considered safe. Focus group participants stated they had not previously worried about the MMR vaccine, but after media coverage of Wakefield's theories, their decision became much more difficult.

> I've got a 13 year old and she's had the MMR but then there was nothing in the papers, any scare so *she was done automatically*.
>
> (emphasis added, N2)

Media coverage was frequently portrayed as a '*catalyst* of concern and worry not only about whether to have MMR but whether previous decisions had been wise' (Petts and Niemeyer 2004: 13). Evans et al. also found that the media publicity 'had raised doubts in the minds of people who had not previously questioned the safety of immunisation' (2001: 906). The media popularised new discursive repertoires, that the MMR vaccine was unsafe and thus influenced the public's sense of identity by challenging their relationships with their GPs and health care workers.

The media play a significant role in constructing discourses which the public use 'to define and understand the world', but as Lewis points out, these discourses are 'not absolute' (Lewis 2001: 84). The main rationales discussed by focus group participants were the fear of autism, fear of the three diseases and concerns about who to trust. All rationales except the fear of autism *existed before* the publication of the 1998 *Lancet* paper. The one rationale used by focus group participants that only exists after the 1998 *Lancet* paper is the fear of autism. Parents develop these rationales based on four main sources of information: media, health professionals, friends and family and their own experiences and knowledge (see Figure 8.4).

Figure 8.4 Where rationales came from

<u>Main rationales</u>   <u>Main sources of information</u>

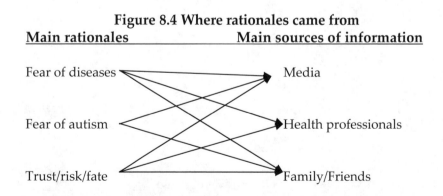

The sources which focus group participants identified as promoting the 'fear of autism' rationale were the media and friends and family.

But the focus groups showed that friends and family also obtained their information from the media. So if one of the main rationales parents used to make their MMR vaccination decision was this 'fear of autism' and if we examine what the main sources were saying to parents, it is clear that the media are the main source for this rationale – both directly and indirectly.

The focus groups suggested parents were considerably affected by the media coverage. All focus group participants (except one, who consumed no news media) reconsidered the safety of the MMR vaccine as a result of media coverage, evidence of a significant 'effect' on the audience. The media coverage told parents not only what to think, but also how to think about the MMR vaccine, that the vaccine might be unsafe and science and governments could not be trusted. The broad pattern of media coverage, the repeated associations with autism and the solution offered by single vaccines, rather than the details of the story, resonated with the audience. Most parents accepted the dominant frame and worried about their MMR vaccine decisions, some modifying their decision or deciding not to vaccinate their children. But by far, most parents negotiated their understanding and trusted health professionals, friends and family more than the media and continued to accept the MMR vaccine.

CHAPTER NINE

Sowing the Seeds of Doubt?

Since Wakefield's *Lancet* research was published in 1998 there has been a search for who to blame and hold responsible for the slow decline in the MMR vaccine uptake. Most frequently the media are blamed for whipping up a frenzy and making a controversy out of a very one-sided scientific debate. Scientists and pro-MMR sources are also blamed for failing to participate consistently in media coverage and promote the safety of the MMR vaccine. They are accused of depending too much on the Department of Health to defend the vaccine. Opposition politicians are blamed for using the MMR debate to score political points and increase their own profiles. Wakefield himself is blamed for using the media and not scientific evidence to promote his theories. The public has incurred no blame. The media are reluctant to accuse their readers of subscribing to certain views, especially when they are reporting these views. The public is also regarded by scientists and science communicators as a victim of sensationalist media coverage. Are they all culpable and are some more culpable than others? The final chapter revisits key themes to reveal how the anti-MMR side achieved more prominence in the media coverage, the effect of this on the audience and the resulting implications for journalists, sources and health educators.

The Prominence of the Anti-MMR Argument

Professional Practices

Evidence that coverage about the MMR vaccine was antagonistic is revealed by considering which participants in the story were the most unhappy with the coverage. Anti-MMR sources were fairly content with the media coverage, yet coverage frustrated and troubled those who promoted the triple vaccine. Various professional practices contributed to the anti-MMR argument being more prominent. Earlier scientific controversies, primarily BSE and GM foods, where 'maverick' scientists were key participants, had a significant influence on how the MMR/autism story was reported. These stories acted as a frame for the MMR/autism controversy. Because of this comparison, the MMR/autism story was regarded as the 'next' scientific controversy, and thus the story quickly moved from the science sections to the news pages and, consequently, from science and health correspondents to general news correspondents. There was no scientific evidence proving the link between the MMR vaccine and autism, but as the MMR/autism story fit the established frame of the government withholding evidence and the impression that the views of a maverick were being suppressed, the story therefore made headline news.

Scientific facts did not figure prominently in the coverage, and instead, the story became a political issue. It became newsworthy because it was a controversy. Applying a controversial and political frame to complex science, health and risk stories increases their news value. In order to broaden its political relevance, the MMR/autism story was framed as part of the larger debate concerning choice in health care as journalists and parents asked for a choice between the MMR and single vaccines. This political frame made it difficult for scientists to participate in the debate. Science and scientists (including all health professionals) appeared infrequently, and they accounted for less than a quarter of all sources, almost half of which were anti-MMR. This story was not so much about science as it was about the politics of health and health care provision.

In order to create a controversial frame, journalists needed to establish Wakefield's claims as credible, and one of the ways they did was to over-balance stories to make his research seem more legitimate and therefore compelling. Half of all stories included both anti- and pro-MMR arguments and an additional third of stories were under-balanced and included only anti-MMR statements and arguments. A typical story featured one source accusing the MMR vaccine of being linked to autism; this was juxtaposed with statements from another source stating its safety, thus giving the appearance of an equally divided debate.

Journalists unfairly balanced the story to make it appear as if an equally divided scientific controversy was exacerbated by the type of sources selected and the presentation of the sources' arguments. One quarter of all sources were scientists, and the remaining sources were parents, politicians, pressure groups, journalists and private health care companies. The stories of parents and pressure groups were told as stories with narratives to follow, either trailing the difficult journey of parents making their vaccination decision or a parent's claim about the cause of their child's autism.

Using parents' claims and accusations about the MMR vaccine's level of safety, which lacked any scientific evidence, raises the complex problem of how to report public opinion when it is in direct opposition to what is accepted scientific fact. This led to significant problems in the reporting and use of expertise in the MMR/autism story. Journalists frequently equated public opinion with scientific arguments, making it appear as if claims made by both sides were equally valid. However, this style of reporting consistently puts science on the defensive and tends to incorrectly equate public *opinion* with scientific expertise.

This research recommends that the media consider the way expertise is reported and proposes the category of 'expert-source'. The CIN (contributory-interactional-none) categories of expertise established by Collins and Evans (2002, 2007) provides a framework to consider the role of expertise in journalism and the reporting of public opinion. By being more forthright about the expertise that a source possesses— contributory, interactional or none— journalists can limit the influence of powerful or elite sources, public relations and pundits who do not have expertise. Journalists thus are able to regain control over (and responsibility for) the stories they are reporting. A more open recognition of who is speaking will contribute to a deliberative democracy and 'opportunities for the credentials and legitimacy of speakers to be questioned and challenged, and for those in turn to be defended and challenges rebutted' (Cottle 2003: 168).

Because of the overt political frame applied to the MMR/autism story, many general news correspondents reported the issue. Their stories were more likely to lead with political statements or emotional narratives of parents than specialist health/science correspondents who were more likely to lead their stories with scientific research. In the same vein, general news correspondents were more likely to depend on the claims of parents to make the link between the MMR vaccine and autism and not refer to scientific evidence. The MMR/autism story was a 'good' and 'easy' story to report for those who had little scientific background knowledge. There was a choice of established frames to choose from (David vs. Goliath/Wakefield vs. rest of science; governments and pharmaceutical companies controlling health care; the fear of children being damaged) and an endless supply of sources (new parents were always making the MMR vaccination decision and therefore new opinions to report and a new audience to target). With so many general news correspondents reporting the MMR/autism story, health and science sources need to make their information, arguments and press material relevant to those with little background knowledge as well as to those journalists they have regular contact with, the specialist correspondents. One press release and one press conference is not adequate to meet the differing needs of journalists with various levels of knowledge and awareness. Providing different styles of information to journalists can potentially broaden relationships to include a variety of journalists, resulting in health and science sources working more closely with general news correspondents, columnists and other specialists.

More noticeable professional practices were used to deliberately make the anti-MMR argument more prominent. The science and health professionals sourced were more frequently anti-MMR and the first sources journalists selected more often espoused the anti-MMR argument. The editorial agendas of certain newspapers promoted anti-MMR arguments and had wider influences on other media outlets because of the pack journalism mentality.

Source In/Activity

In addition to the actions and attitudes of journalists, sources' practices also led to the coverage being more anti- than pro-MMR. Pro-MMR scientific sources abdicated responsibility to the Department of Health and depended on them to promote and defend the MMR vaccine. But because of the decreased level of trust in government agencies arising from earlier scientific controversies, journalists were sceptical of the DoH, branding them 'heavy-handed' or untrustworthy. In addition, as health and science sources took exactly the same position as the DoH, their statements were not newsworthy, as journalists already had the argument 'MMR is safe' from the DoH. Journalists needed newsworthy copy, and sources who could provide newsworthy material different from the DoH were more likely to receive coverage than if they simply repeated the government message.

The pro-MMR message was more complex and thus more difficult to argue in a short period. 'MMR is the safest way to vaccinate your child' was a difficult argument to make in 1 or 2 sentences compared to the short and succinct 'MMR is unsafe, it might be linked to autism'. Statements challenging safety were more easily reported than the detailed statements as to why the MMR vaccine was safe. The job of the DoH and official health sources is to promote public health messages, but this is likely in the future to become more challenging for a number of reasons. Public relations skills are now more ubiquitous, health care issues are more important in an aging population, private health care is now an option for more and more of the population and media competition is more ruthless.

The MMR/autism story illustrates how UK scientists have learned little about dealing with earlier scientific controversies. In the past, scientists have been reluctant to participate in debates where science stories have evolved into stories involving more than just science. But if scientists leave ethical or controversial debates only to those without scientific expertise and knowledge, there will be an absence of science in these decisions, thus affecting the tone of the debate. The UK science community needs to consider how it will handle future mavericks (on 9 December 2006 the UK science magazine *New Scientist* published a series of articles entitled 'Lone Voices' in an attempt to progress the debate about how the UK scientific community deals with 'maverick' scientists). The MMR/autism story reveals the power of the media to influence public health, and sources acknowledge there is growing evidence of the power and responsibility the media can wield in media health debates. In 2004 Richard Horton, editor of *The Lancet,* accepted that his actions played a part in the MMR/autism controversy (Horton 2004a) and that medical journals are influential in medical and health stories and controversies. In June 2004 Mike Fitzpatrick, a general practitioner and father of an autistic child, published an expose of the science and fiction behind the MMR vaccine controversy. Horton soon followed with a treatise on the controversy published in September 2004.

In the past few years organisations like the Science Media Centre (SMC) have been created to provide the media with scientists who have been trained to speak to the media and are relevant to the scientific debate being reported. They encourage scientists to talk to the media, especially during controversies, and provide background briefings on key issues to improve how science and health is reported.

The need for an organisation like the SMC and its success has led to it being copied in other countries (established in Australia and soon to open in New Zealand and South Africa).

The influence of public relations on scientists and science/medical journals also contributed to how the story became anti-MMR. Wakefield's PR efforts demonstrate the significant impact an individual can have on the way a story is reported, demonstrating how an individual can radically influence media coverage and secure 'definitional advantage' (Cottle 2003: 7). Accusations of sensationalising science and health stories, personalising complex issues or emphasising maverick views have traditionally been made of the mainstream media, but these charges can now also be levelled against medical journals. *Lancet* editor Richard Horton (2004a) acknowledges medical journals now employ these methods for much the same reason as mainstream media, to increase circulation and advertising revenue. Whilst previous research examined the impact of medical and scientific journal press releases (for example, Entwistle 1995), research now needs to consider the wider range of public relations tactics employed by medical and scientific journals.

The scientific community is beginning to address its role and responsibilities in the communication of research. The Royal Society addressed 'the extent to which the public interest is considered by the research community in science, engineering and technology in relation to the communication of research results'. This acknowledged that science and health journals play a large role in the type of issues that are covered in the mainstream media (Royal Society 2006: 7). The report concluded that the research community had two main responsibilities: to provide accurate assessments of the potential implications to the public and to ensure 'the timely and appropriate communication to the public of results if such communication is in the public interest (ibid.: 5).

A relatively new factor to consider when looking at why medical issues receive coverage is the role of private health care. Spending on private health care continues to rise alongside the government's emphasis on the patient as a consumer in the NHS. The MMR/autism story illustrates the problems private health care PR can contribute to a public health issue because of their competition for customers/audiences. In the MMR/autism story, private health care PR influenced how the story was reported, as they provided easy access to anti-MMR parents and good visual backdrops for television news reports.

Sowing the Seeds of Doubt

Media coverage led parents to question the safety of the MMR vaccine and prompted them to worry and about a vaccine they were previously not worried about.

> The thing is though, the seeds are sown and then people just start thinking on the down side of it...I had no problem with it at all until that seed was sown.
>
> (M2)

> **V3:** But there's always an element of truth whatever you read, there's always an element of truth in it, (media's) not based on complete fabrication isn't it? (There's) got to be an element of truth somewhere along the line. So therefore that's what I think you make your decision on...
> **V1:** It's (media coverage) enough to sow the seeds of doubt.
> **V3:** Yes, exactly, the element of truth just starts you off.

When 'new' stories hit the news, the media initiate conversations; they 'set the agenda'. When the media report new ideas they tell the public 'what to think about'. The difference between telling the public to think *about* an issue rather than what *to* think of an issue is blurred when new stories are reported. By getting people to think *about* the MMR vaccine, the media set the scene for a change in uptake rates. The media have an influential and important role when reporting new scientific stories (Kitzinger 2004 and Hornig-Priest 1999). In the case of the MMR/autism story, media coverage introduced the parents to the idea that the triple vaccine might be unsafe. For example, one vaccinating parent describes that she worried *because of* the media coverage.

> I think because there are more headlines around I think I would've asked more questions at this point than I did back then (pre-1998).
>
> (V7)

The media coverage prompted parents to worry, but ultimately, the audience did not blindly consume the dominant frame—their responses were mediated by other factors. The MMR vaccine uptake fell by approximately 12%, with the majority of parents continuing to choose the MMR vaccine. These pro-MMR parents used their own experiences and knowledge to make their vaccination decision. Evidence from focus groups and the media analysis found that parents who vaccinated with the MMR vaccine were convinced by the immunisation decisions of people they respected, asking their GPs, friends and family if their children had had the vaccine. Many parents also had direct experience of the MMR vaccine, as they had vaccinated their older children.

The reason why the coverage 'sowed the seeds of doubt' was because of the power of association: the impact of balance and the strength of narratives all led to the MMR/autism link being a credible issue to consider. Much research using agenda-setting theory finds that 'the media can be a powerful influence on what audiences believe and what is thought to be legitimate or desirable' (Philo 1999: 287). Whilst journalists did not necessarily endorse Wakefield's claims, the sheer repetition of the idea that the MMR vaccine might be linked to autism appears to have influenced public understanding of this issue. One powerful way in which the media can influence people is by establishing 'associations' (Kitzinger 1999b, Lewis 1991, 2001). Both the surveys and the focus groups found the public had clearly associated the MMR vaccine with autism. What also lingered in the public's mind was the traditional 'balanced' approach taken by many reports. The public was left with the impression of an equally divided body of research and was largely unaware that Wakefield was one of very few scientists claiming a link between the MMR vaccine and autism.

What was not in the media coverage also influenced audience reception of this story. The public learned 'facts' about the MMR vaccine, suggesting the power of the media to inform and create associations. One of the facts they did not learn, because it was not reported in the media, was the risk of measles, mumps or rubella. The media paid more attention to the supposed risks of the vaccine and little attention to research into the causes of autism or the risks of the three diseases, and as a consequence parents knew little about these issues. They knew about the MMR/autism link but little detail beyond this.

Parents were not interested in the merits of the scientific evidence or argument; they wanted to be told what to do. They asked opinion leaders (GPs, health visitors, midwives, family and friends) whether they had their children vaccinated with the MMR vaccine, but their questions stopped there—they did not ask *why* they had made these decisions. Focus group participants stated they wanted access to more scientific information, but when they had the chance to ask health professionals questions, they frequently only asked if they had given the MMR vaccine to their child. They wanted someone to make the MMR vaccination decision for them and for someone else to take the responsibility in case something went wrong. This attitude contrasts with the Labour government's idea of a reflexive and educated health consumer making their own choices in health care and instead reveals that the public continues to depend on health professionals' opinions and expertise.

Is the Answer More Science?

One problem for future health controversies is the dichotomy between what audiences say they want in order to make their own decisions about their health and the reality of how they make these decisions. In reflecting on how they made their MMR decisions, focus group participants suggested ways to improve the type of information they wanted and how it should be communicated. Interestingly, the suggestions only concerned ways for the media and health professionals to improve: they did not refer to their own actions or the information provided by their friends and family. In focus groups, participants were quick to call for *more* science in media coverage. The media analysis found scientific facts did not dominate coverage, but they were there; so if these audiences scoured the media and read entire articles in detail, they would find some of the information they requested was already in the coverage. But the public is more likely to remember headlines (van Dijk 1991), and participants admitted this when they requested that key information *be in the headlines* (e.g., 'Wakefield's study only on 12 children'), not for it just to be in the media.

In order to improve the communication of the pro-MMR side of the debate, participants argued that they wanted to hear more science and from a wider range of sources. Focus group participants claimed they wanted information and expertise in order to make decisions about their child's health. Parents consistently stated they wanted and trusted information from their GPs and health professionals. The crucial point was that parents wanted information directly from health professionals and not via the media. This might appear to justify the decisions by the DoH to avoid the media and concentrate on using GPs and health professionals to promote the MMR vaccine. Nonetheless, MMR uptake did drop, thus media coverage was a problem. It was a mistake for scientific and medical organisations to ignore media coverage and assume people would go to their GPs for advice. The media coverage caused the focus group participants to worry about the MMR vaccine, which led them to turn to a variety of sources for advice and information, but they also wanted to see the MMR vaccine defended and promoted more actively in the media.

Focus group participants wanted personal contact with their GPs to help make this decision and not leaflets or promotional material which might empower them to make the decision on their own. Although focus group participants stated significant worries about autism, none of them made an effort to find out more about the likely causes or general information about the disorder, as one focus group explained:

> **TB:** Has it made you want to find out more about autism, like you worry about it?
> **V5:** No, not for me.
> **V4:** Not everything's a great worry or autism.
> **V5:** Autism. I don't particularly want to find out about autism, it hasn't made me interested.
> **V4:** I'm too lazy I think.
> **V5:** Too many other things to do.

If parents state they want more information yet do not take the opportunity or time to absorb this information, it is hard for health professionals or scientists to prepare appropriate materials. The assumption that audiences want more scientific evidence even when the audience claims this is what they want is sometimes in direct opposition to what audiences use when making decisions. Although parents stated that they would be convinced by 'facts', many times parents' fact were incomplete or incorrect. They were more likely to remember the *story* of the MMR vaccine, including the accounts of damaged children and their exhausted and frustrated parents trying to uncover the truth.

The MMR/autism story is one of an increasing number of stories that depict the patient as consumer, now a dominant theme in contemporary health coverage in the UK. The demand for single vaccines, not supported by any scientific evidence, feeds into this idea of choice for 'patient-consumers' and was a recurring theme. The effect of this rise of consumerism in medical coverage 'has challenged the power of doctors to make decisions about patient care' (Lupton 1998:

196). When patients become consumers, they are expected and expect to take more control of the 'product' they 'purchase' and will then inform themselves. One of the impacts of the rise of consumerism in medicine is a public which has become 'more demanding, less deferential…more knowledgeable through internet and media (and where) information is no longer a secret weapon of the profession' (Ham and Alberti 2002: 840). But whether or not patients want this responsibility should not be assumed. Patients might not have the skills to find this information or might have difficult relationships with their general practitioners and thus 'many patients do not want to take responsibility or seek out information for themselves – they are more happy to trust their health professionals and leave decisions to them' (Henwood et al. 2004: 88). The idea of the patient-consumer, seeking out extra information and taking more responsibility for their own health decisions can lead to decisions that are not what mainstream science would recommend. If the NHS and governments want the public to become more responsible for making health care decisions, then they need to acknowledge that these decisions might not be what they would advocate.

The MMR Vaccine and Reporting Science, Health and Risks

The era of the 'public understanding of science' where the unknowing public is taught scientific facts in order for people to make decisions has now been replaced by a belief in 'science in society', where the public plays a more active role in science. At the same time, journalism is also becoming more democratic with the rise of citizen journalism and user-generated content. If science and journalism are both becoming more democratised and audience-led, what impact will this have on the reporting of science, health and risk stories? The MMR/autism story demonstrates the powerful influence non-specialist journalists and citizens, those who lack expertise or knowledge, can have on a complex science story which has potentially wide-ranging health implications. Journalism is central to 'successful functioning of democratic societies' and creates space for a dialogue between politicians and the public (Lewis and Wahl-Jorgensen 2005: 99). But if science becomes more democratised, is it the media's job to 'create a space for dialogue between scientists and the public'? The media does create spaces for dialogues but other factors influence the level and type of dialogue. News values influence which dialogues appear in the media and which frames are attached to them. This can mean a science dialogue, in the quest to make it appealing to the broadest possible audience, is devoid of scientific evidence and fact. Making science or health stories relevant can impede the potential usefulness of the dialogue.

Is it still relevant to ask questions about reporting the MMR/autism story? MMR vaccination rates have increased slowly and only stand at 84%, still well below the 96% coverage achieved in 1995, confirming that 'public concern and policy attention rises and falls in response to shifts in media coverage (rather than changes in the actual size of the problem in the real world)' (Kitzinger 2004: 14). There are signs this story is making inroads in other countries. In the summer of 2004 the *Washington Post* published an article about the MMR vaccine controversy and the implications for American children and parents, and with Wakefield based in the USA, his efforts are more likely have an effect where he is based.

The MMR/autism story tapped into strong feelings about distrusting science, children and family life and these issues are now being raised in more recent vaccine stories. On 15 March 2004 the *Daily Mail* reported another vaccine might be linked to autism, this time the Diphtheria-Tetanus-Pertussis vaccine (DTP). The reporting was similar to the MMR/autism story. The story, published on page 41, begins 'A controversial vaccination…'. Coverage replicates that found in the MMR/autism story with the language emphasising the vaccine as dangerous. The first three sources all raise problems with the DTP vaccine and the Department of Health's response is relegated to the penultimate paragraph.

Will the MMR/autism story ever come to an end? Will there be scientific or policy developments which will provide 'closure' or will media values and practices continue to be the crucial factor in determining whether this story is covered? Many specialist health and science correspondents have tired of this story, but general news correspondents continue to regard the MMR/autism story as newsworthy. Nonetheless, there will be more health and science stories in the future where the balance of evidence will be problematic and where public health will be affected. Journalists, sources and the audience can all learn from how the MMR/autism story has unfolded and the implications for the way future science, health and risk stories are reported.

Notes

Chapter One

1   Herd immunity is '(w)hen vaccine levels are at a high level in a community, the risk of disease is so low that even those who are not immune are unlikely to be affected' (Fitzpatrick 2004: 12). The World Health Organisation recommends this level to be 95%.

2   This financial incentive came in for criticism in 2002 when some parents tried to argue GPs were encouraging vaccinations not because of the health of children, but because of these 'bonuses'. The incentive remains and has been effectively ignored by the media since the height of the media attention in 2002.

3   The cost varies from clinic to clinic and has increased from under £200 in the late 1990s to closer to £400 in 2006.

4   This is often done purposely in another country and then UK GPs are obliged to offer the other vaccines separately.

5   All MMR uptake statistics in the book are from the Health Protection Authority (formerly Public Health Laboratory Service) website www.hpa.org.uk/infections/topics_az/vaccination/vac_coverage.htm. The statistics are measured by the number of children who had received the vaccine by their second birthday. The government admits that the measuring system is not perfect as it does not measure those vaccinated after their second birthday, nor children who have had single vaccines, nor does the system keep track of children who move out of their initial assessment area. Scientists continue to research improved ways of collecting these statistics.

6   Available at http://briandeer.com/wakefield/royal-video.htm (Accessed March 2007).

7   UK national newspapers include those available on LexisNexis, US newspapers include *USA Today, Wall Street Journal, New York Times, Los Angeles Times, Washington Post, New York Daily News*. England and Wales vaccination rates from Health Protection Agency, USA vaccination rates from the Centers for Disease Control – see footnote 5.

8   Hence there are no references to cite.

9   The article was to be published in April 2002 but was pre-published on the internet in February following high demand after the *Panorama* programme was aired. *Molecular Pathology* has since ceased to exist. In January 2004 this journal with a small circulation was 'folded into' its parent journal, the *Journal of Clinical Pathology*. http://jcp.bmjjournals.com/

10 These measles outbreaks occurred in parts of London inhabited by many middle-class journalists, perhaps part of the reason why they attracted so much attention.

11   One of the main private providers of single vaccines in the UK.

12   The Center is part of the Good News Doctor Foundation, which describes itself as 'A Christian ministry that provides hope and information on how to eat better, feel better, and minister more effectively as a result of a biblically based, healthy lifestyle.' www.gnd.org

13   In Japan, between 1994 and 1999, 85 people died from measles after the MMR vaccine was withdrawn in 1993 after the strain of mumps virus (Urabe) used in the vaccine caused cases of aseptic mumps viral meningitis. Since then Japan has used single measles and rubella vaccines. Research found increases in incidence of autism even when the MMR vaccine was withdrawn (Honda et al. 2005).

14   See, for instance: Bandolier (2002), Dales et al. (2001), DeWilde et al. (2001), Donald and Muthu (2002), Kaye et al. (2001), Madsen et al. (2002), Patja et al. (2002), Peltola et al. (1998), Peltola et al. (1994), Taylor et al. (1999) and Taylor et al. (2002).

15   That autism is one of the most heritable psychiatric conditions, see, for instance, Gillberg, C. (1983) 'Identical Triplets with Infantile Autism and the Fragile–X Syndrome' *British Journal of Psychiatry*. 143:256–260 or Bailey, A., LeCouteur, A., Gottesman, I. and Bolton, P. (1995) 'Autism as a Strongly Genetic Disorder: Evidence from a British Twin Study' *Psychological Medicine*. 25: 63–77. For reviews of autism and its suspected causes see Rinehart, N.J., Bradshaw, J.L., Brereton, A.V. and Tonge, B.J. (2002) 'A Clinical and Neurobehavioural Review of High-Functioning Autism and Asperger's Disorder' *Australian and New Zealand Journal of Psychiatry*. 36:762–770; Yang, M.S., Gill, M. (2007) 'A review of gene linkage, association and expression studies in autism and an assessment of convergent evidence' *International Journal of Developmental Neuroscience*. 25: 69–85. Many thanks to Dr. Chris Ashwin for his advice on this issue.

16   Research into the media and the MMR vaccine *before* Wakefield made the MMR/autism link argued that the media were not a reason for refusal (Roberts et al. 1995). However, the vaccine had received little publicity in the national media at this point (see Table 1.1, page 6), thus this finding should not be understood to imply that the media had no impact. The media were also not mentioned in a 1994 *BMJ* article examining parental myths about immunisation. Begg et al. (1998) argued it was more important to try to influence official sources like the Department of Health, immunisation advisory clinics, vaccine manufacturers, parents and grandparents.

17   This legal case was led by solicitor Richard Barr, who, as Fitzpatrick (2004a) outlines, first came to public attention in the late 1980s after pursuing compensation for patients who claimed they had suffered damaging side effects from the anti-inflammatory drug Opren. Barr has also taken up a number of high profile medical cases (what would be labelled as 'class-action suits' in the USA); alleged victims from organophosphates in farming, ex-soldiers suffering from Gulf War Syndrome and the families who claim their children have been damaged by vaccines.

18   See www.briandeer.com.

19   They have since expanded to include campaigning for children whom parents claim were damaged from other vaccines.

20 Interview with author.

21 The increase in mumps cases was predicted by the HPA (outlined in a press statement issued 2 November 2004, Available at http://www.hpa.org.uk/ hpa/news/ articles/press_releases/2004/041102_mumps.htm. In spring 2006 the UK had its first death from measles since the introduction of the MMR vaccine. The 14 year old was immuno-suppressed and unable to have the MMR vaccine. Whether or not more widespread herd immunity would have protected the child is difficult to prove. Previous to this, no immuno-suppressed children have died since the introduction of the MMR vaccine.

22 See www.hpa.org.uk

23 Different statistics exist on the rate of decline, thse statistics are from Baker 2003 and Begg et al. 1998, who estimate the rate fell from 81% to 31%. Nonetheless, the drop was significant.

24 Previous research does not analyse whether the parents were against *all* vaccines or just vocal opponents of the pertussis vaccine. This is relevant as the group campaigning against the MMR vaccine, Justice, Awareness and Basic Support (JABS), state they are not anti-vaccine but against all vaccines which damage children, hence their support for single measles, mumps and rubella vaccines.

25 In 2002 broadsheets and tabloids were yet to change traditional formats. All tabloid style papers in the sample were popular papers; therefore the terms 'broadsheets' and 'tabloids' are used.

26 www.bbc.co.uk/radio4/today. In 2002 the *Today* programme website typically included 12-15 stories per day. When asked how it was decided which stories would be included, the *Today* programme responded that they simply selected the 'significant' stories. The entire programme is now online.

27 At the time, I was told by Visceral that Wakefield was primarily working in the USA and therefore not available for interviews. Visceral offered to forward any emails to Wakefield but I did not take up this offer as I could not be assured the emails would be answered by Wakefield. My request for an interview was further exacerbated when I was invited to participate in a televised debate that followed a drama about the MMR/autism story. Entitled 'Hear the Silence' this two hour drama starred Juliet Stephenson and was sympathetic to Wakefield and his views. In the debate I was physically placed in the 'pro-MMR' camp even though I informed the producers I was there to discuss my research and was not arguing for or against the MMR vaccine. At the recording of the programme, I approached Robert Sawyer, chief executive of Visceral, before the debate, and repeated my request for an interview with Wakefield, who was standing 10 feet from me but surrounded by people. Sawyer said this was fine and to send him a list of questions in an email, and when I stated I would rather interview him quickly over the telephone, he excused himself from the conversation. Wakefield was unapproachable before and after the debate as he had a circle of supporters around him and was not easily approached.

Chapter Two

1   From conversations with PHLS/HPA and DoH personnel.

2   Only one article (*Guardian* 2 February 2002) referred to London's historically low vaccination rate due to its mobile population and number of immigrants, even though my own interviews revealed the DoH had consistently reminded journalists of this fact.

3   In the 1990s the 'Alan Sokal' experiments exposed the problems of peer review in the humanities, specifically cultural studies. Sokal (1996) wrote the article 'Transgressing the Boundaries: Toward a Transformative Hermeneutics of Quantum Gravity' to satirise the subjective/post-modern turn in intellecutal and political academe. His paper was a fallacy but passed the peer review process for the journal *Social Text*. For further explanation on how this story evolved, see his website: www.physics.nyu.edu/faculty/sokal/.

4   For example, *Lancet* editor Richard Horton writes of pharmaceutical companies increasing use of ghostwriters to publish supportive research in medical journals, estimating that half of articles in journals come from those writing on behalf of the pharmaceutical industry (Horton 2004a), see also Jacky Law's (2006) expose of global pharmaceutical companies.

5   From interviews with scientists and journalists.

6   See Fitzpatrick (2004: 140-141) for explanation as to why this claim is erroneous.

7   See, for instance, his publication in the small journal *Molecular Pathology* (Uhlmann et al. 2002) or in the *Israeli Medical Association Journal* (Wakefield and Montgomery 1999).

8   Of course, the problem is that Wakefield made his accusations about the MMR vaccine and his proposed solution, single vaccines, in the subsequent press conference, not in the paper itself. Thus Horton could honestly state that *The Lancet* article did not argue the MMR vaccine was unsafe. The article itself did not assert causality, but as the Royal Free had made a video press release where Wakefield stated single vaccines should be available on the NHS, then Horton was most likely aware of the problems the article was likely to raise.

9   An 'Agony Aunt' answers letters from readers about a variety of personal issues. Dr. Miriam Stoppard is different from most Agony Aunts as she is a qualified General Practitioner, so most of her questions are medically-related. Most Agony Aunts are unqualified and answer emotional/relationship queries.

Chapter Three

1   As discussed in Chapter 1, this disassociation was in light of revelations that there might be a conflict of interest as Wakefield received funding from the Legal Services Commission to look into the potential link between the MMR vaccination and autism at the same time as he published the 1998 *Lancet* paper.

2   This was a significant theme in the Channel 5 drama 'Hear the Silence'.

3 Fitzpatrick discusses the increase in autism and raises the issues about the increase in awareness versus the actual increase in cases of autism (2004: 74-77). See also Footnote 15 Chapter 1.

4 Although Channel 5 has raised the idea that television news should abandon its impartiality and take sides and provide news with an open bias, similar to that produced by the American 'Fox' television network (see for example Jones 2003).

5 The Hutton inquiry was initiated after the death of Dr. David Kelly, an anonymous source (and employee of the Ministry of Defence) for *Today* programme presenter Andrew Gilligan. Gilligan reported that an anonymous source (reportedly Kelly) claimed the Labour government had deliberately exaggerated the threat of Iraq's so-called weapons of mass destruction. Kelly's name was linked as the possible anonymous source and Kelly admitted he had met with Gilligan and other BBC journalists to provide off-the-record briefs. Kelly's body was found near his home soon after the revelations that he might be the anonymous source. Lord Hutton was asked to carry out an inquiry into the matter and his published report exonerated the government and placed all of the blame on the BBC, leading to the director-general's and chairman's resignations.

6 One of the earliest studies examining the relationship between science coverage and public opinion found that the appearance of a dispute often works to benefit *opponents* of technology (see Mazur 1981).

7 In the subsequent years since the initial interest in Leo Blair's vaccination status this story has infrequently reappeared. It appears the story's newsworthy value was linked to Leo's being at vaccination age.

8 For an explanation of focus group labels see beginning of Chapter 8.

9 The MMR/autism story challenges previous findings which conclude commercial considerations affect coverage, for if the related product is not advertised in the mainstream media, as is the case for vaccines, then media coverage is not affected. This finding might be different in the USA, where direct-to-consumer advertising is officially permitted and more widespread.

Chapter Four

1 When we made this criticism about balance in our *Towards a Better Map* report, journalists denounced our finding. John Mason of the *Financial Times* argued broadcasters had a 'legal duty to be impartial' and defended their practice of balancing Wakefield's evidence with the rest of science.

2 My own research can be criticised for using the same binary oppositions that journalists use as I often refer to the pro- and anti-MMR 'sides'. I am reflecting what is in the media rather than agreeing with the way the media reduces this complex debate.

3 As Alasuutari (1999) argues, '(c)overage is also influenced by everyday journalistic practices (including practical constraints such as deadlines and word limits) and how journalists envisage their audiences' (in Davidson et al. 2004: 21).

4 Without doing any media analysis, scientists had correctly hypothesised that the media had emphasised anti-MMR parents, and as they stated, 'the vast majority

(of parents) will go on to have their child immunised with MMR' (Ramsay et al. 2002: 916).

5   In interviews, the sources, including the DoH, recommended independent scientists to journalists but none of these scientists had made much of an impression with the journalists interviewed.

6   Dearing (1994) makes a similar point in his research – sources were frustrated that journalists felt balance was always 'desirable'.

Chapter Five

1   Includes scientists, doctors, nurses, health visitors.

2   Includes, for example, teachers, headteachers, celebrities.

3   As Chapter 1 explained, the Conservative party introduced the MMR vaccine in 1988 and had been supportive of the triple jab in the subsequent period. In 2001-2002 the Tory party changed their stance and instead supported the 'right' for parents to choose between the MMR vaccine and single vaccines on the NHS.

4   See, for example, 10 February 2002 *Sunday Times* 'Dr Maverick sticks to his guns' by Rosie Waterhouse.

5   *Private Eye* is a political satirical magazine issued weekly in the UK.

6   Hornby wrote an almost verbatim copy of the article that appeared the next day in the *Daily Mail*.

7   The National Autistic Society represents both parents who believe the MMR caused their child's autism and those who do not; consequently, its official view is fairly ambiguous.

8   In September 2004 a pro-MMR parent (not health professional) appeared on Radio 5 Live phone-in arguing on behalf of the MMR vaccine and claimed to be part of a wider group supporting the MMR vaccine. The group was not named and has not had a significant media impact.

9   This was revealed by the *Daily Mail* on 17 June 2002 'Dr Wakefield...(w)orking with the Direct Health clinic in London...'. Kathryn Durnford was the representative during this period and went on to become managing director of a private provider of single vaccines, Healthcare UK. Their website reads 'Healthchoice UK is a primary health care group established to provide the consumer with greater health care choice for themselves and their family. We bring together an indepth knowledge of current medicinal thinking and efficient healthcare service'. www.healthchoiceuk.co.uk/ Accessed 24 April 2007

Chapter Six

1   Fitzpatrick agrees that doctors and scientists who wanted to challenge Wakefield's claims would only 'provide even more publicity for the anti-MMR campaign' (2004: 36).

2   Miller and Reilly (1995: 318) make a similar point in relation to the food industry and so-called maverick scientists.

3   Some with more success than others. In September 2004 the Welsh arm of the BMA organised for a young girl to give her own views as part of an anti-smoking presentation to the Welsh Assembly. The Welsh Assembly rejected their request to include this young girl's opinions stating the BMA would be better to stick to their scientific arguments than rely on second-rate publicity. It appears that scientists can't win!

4   Lynda Lee Potter was a *Daily Mail* columnist.

5   The 'MMR: The Facts' campaign continues today, see www.mmrthefacts.nhs.uk. (Accessed July 2007)

6   As Chapter 1 explains, when the vaccination rates for the pertussis vaccine fell from 80% to 30%.

Chapter Seven

1   A version of this chapter first appeared in *Journalism Studies* (Boyce 2007). Kind thanks and appreciation to its editor for permission to reprint a version of the article.

2   The author has participated in a series of workshops with Collins and Evans to help develop the CIN theory of expertise.

3   From an interview with the author.

4   Collins and Evans give the example of estimating the inflation rate where 'forecasts are based on masses of historical data, a first class understanding of economics, and complex computer models, but they can still get it wrong, sometimes very wrong and they often disagree markedly' (2007).

Chapter Eight

1   The surveys were conducted by Research and Marketing Ltd in Cardiff, Wales, UK. 1035 subjects were surveyed in April and 1037 surveyed in October. The samples were weighted to be nationally representative in terms of gender, age and social class.

2   This measurement includes only the first MMR vaccine and not the booster. See www.hpa.gov.uk and www.wales.gov.uk/statistics for complete immunisation statistics. All statistics taken from these two websites. Vaccination uptake rates are affected by geography, with low rates in pockets of the UK and high rates in the majority of the country. Thus the focus group participants reflect the geography of the Cardiff area, where the uptake rate is 85%, higher than the national average (see: http://new.wales.gov.uk/legacy_en/keypubstatistics for wales/content/publication/health). In Wales the uptake rate was as high as 92% in the mid-1990s but in 2002-2003 it fell to 81%, the lowest since its introduction.

3   Petts and Niemeyer (2004) also found similarly low use of the internet for parents seeking information about the MMR vaccine.

4   This question is based on October results only. The first survey only separated science education into 'any' and 'none' and results were not specific enough so the categories were modified in the second survey.

5   She had previously worked for the scientist Professor John O'Leary, who has published papers with Wakefield.

6   There were so few other media images available of autistic children or adults and parents rarely mentioned other cultural images of autism. In this period there were few other significant representations of autism in British culture and this was one of the frustrations discussed in the interview with the publicity officer at the National Autistic Society. Since the 2002 research sample, there have been a number of television documentaries on terrestrial and digital channels discussing autism and these were occasionally referred to in focus groups.

7   Wakefield and JABS do not discuss other multiple vaccines as possibly 'overwhelming' the immune system – such as the DPT vaccine (diphtheria, pertussis and tetanus), which is also a triple vaccine given at the age of one as being of particular concern. Nor have the media picked up on this parallel story.

8   Not to be forgotten is John Gummer's attempt to assuage fears about beef by feeding his children burgers during the BSE crisis, which appeared to backfire.

Bibliography

Albaek, E., Christiansen, P.M. and Togeby, L. (2003) 'Experts in the mass media: Researchers as sources in Danish daily newspapers, 1961-2001', *Journalism and Mass Communication Quarterly*, 80(4): 937-948.

Allan, S. (2002) *Media, Risk, and Science*. Berkshire: Open University Press.

Alterman, E. (1992) *Sound and Fury*. New York: Harper Collins Publishers.

Anderson, A. (1993) 'Source-media relations: The production of the environmental agenda' in Hansen, A. (ed.) *The Mass Media and Environmental Issues*. Leicester: Leicester University Press.

Anke, M., Jong-van den Berg, L., Haaijer-Ruskamp, F., Willems, J. and Tromp, T. (1994) 'Medical journalists and expert sources on medicines', *Public Understanding of Science*, 3: 309-321.

Baker, J.P. (2003) 'The Pertussis Vaccine Controversy in Great Britain, 1974-1986', *Vaccine*, 21: 4003-4010.

Bandolier (2002) 'MMR Vaccination'. www.jr2.ox.ac.uk/bandolier/ band84/MMR.html (accessed March 2007).

Beck, U. (1992) *Risk Society*. London: Sage.

Begg, N., Ramsay, M., White, J. and Bozoky, Z. (1998) 'Media dents confidence in MMR vaccine', *British Medical Journal*, 316 (7130): 516.

Bell, A. (1991) *The Language of News Media*. Blackwell: Oxford.

Bell, A. (1994) 'Media (mis)communication on the science of climate change', *Public Understanding of Science*, 3: 259-275.

Bennett, W.L., et al. (1985) 'Toward a new political narrative', *Journal of Communication*, 35: 156-171.

Berkowitz, D. and TerKeurst, J.V. (1999) 'Community as interpretive community: Rethinking the journalist-source relationship', *Journal of Communication*, Summer: 125-136.

Bishop, R. (2001) 'News media, heal thyselves: Sourcing patterns in news sources about news media performance', *Journal of Communication Inquiry*, 25(1): 22-37.

Bosman, J. (2006) 'Reporters find science journals harder to trust, but not easy to verify', *New York Times*, February 13. Business Section p. C-1.

Bourdieu, P. (1996) *On Television*. New York: The New Press.

Boyce, T. (2007) 'Journalism and expertise', *Journalism Studies*, 7(6): 889-907.

Boyce, T., Lewis, J. and Kitzinger, J. (2007) *Science is Everyday News: Media Trends Report to the Office of Science and Innovation.* Cardiff: Cardiff School of Journalism, Media and Cultural Studies.

Boyd-Barrett, O., Seymour-Ure, C. and Tunstall, J. (eds.) (1977) *Studies on the Press.* Cardiff: HMO.

Boynton, P. (2002) 'Sexperts gag at kebab korrelation', *New Scientist,* May 18: 51.

British Medical Association (2003) *Childhood Immunisation: A Guide for Healthcare Professionals.* London: BMA Board of Science and Education.

Brookes, R. (2000) 'Tabloidisation, media panics and mad cow disease' in Sparks, C. and Tulloch, J. (eds.) *Tabloid Tales: Global Debates Over Media Standards.* Oxford: Rowman and Littlefield.

Brosius, H. and Weimann, G. (1994) 'Who sets the agenda: Agenda-setting as a two-step flow', *International Journal of Public Opinion Research,* 6(4): 323-341.

Brown, J.D. and Walsh-Childers, K. (2002) 'Effects of media on personal and public health' in Bryant, J. and Zillman, D. (eds). *Media Effects: Advances in Theory and Research.* Hillsdale, NJ: Lawrence Erlbaum Associates

Chapman, S. and Lupton, D. (1995) 'The fight for public health', *British Journal of Medicine,* 270.

Chen, R.T. and Stefano, F. (1998) 'Vaccine adverse events: Causal or coincidental?', *The Lancet,* 351: 611-612.

Clayton, A., Hancock-Beaulieu, M. and Meadows, J. (1993) 'Change and continuity in the reporting of science and technology: A study of *The Times* and the *Guardian*', *Public Understanding of Science,* 2: 225-234.

Clements, C.J. and Ratzan, S. (2003) 'Misled and confused? Telling the public about MMR vaccine safety', *Journal of Medical Ethics,* 29: 22-26.

Cohen, B. (1963) *The Press and Foreign Policy.* Princeton, New Jersey: Princeton University Press.

Coleman, C. (1995) 'Science, technology and risk coverage of a community conflict', *Media, Culture and Society,* 17: 65-79.

Collins, H. and Evans, R. (2002) 'The third wave of science studies: Studies of expertise and experiences', *Social Studies of Science,* 32(2): 235-296.

Collins, H. and Evans, R. (2007) *Rethinking Expertise.* Chicago: University of Chicago Press.

Condit, C. (1989) 'The rhetorical limits of polysemy', *Critical Studies in Mass Communication,* 6: 103-122.

Conrad, P. (1999) 'Uses of expertise: Sources, quotes and voice in the reporting of genetics in the news', *Public Understanding of Science,* 8: 285-302.

Corner, J. and Richardson, K. (1993) 'Environmental communication and the contingency of meaning: A research note' in Hansen, A. (ed.) *The Mass Media and Environmental Issues.* Leicester: Leicester University Press.

Cottle, S. (1998) 'Ulrich Beck, "risk society" and the media', *European Journal of Communication,* 13(1): 5-32.

Cottle, S. (2000) 'TV news, lay voices and the visualisation of environmental risks' in Allan, S., Adam, B. and Carter, C. (eds.) *Environmental Risks and the Media*. London: Routledge.

Cottle, S. (2003) 'TV journalism and deliberative democracy: Mediating communicative action' in Cottle, S. (ed.) *News, Public Relations and Power*. London: Sage.

Cracknell, J. (1993) 'Issue arenas, pressure groups and environmental agendas' in Hansen, A. (ed.) *The Mass Media and Environmental Issues*. Leicester: Leicester University Press.

Croteau, D. and Hoynes, W. (1994) *By Invitation Only: How the Media Limit Political Debate*. Monroe, ME: Common Courage Press.

Crouse, T. (1974) *Boys on the Bus*. New York: Ballantine.

Cunningham, B. (2003) 'Re-thinking objectivity', *Columbia Journalism Review*, 42(2): 24-32.

Dales, L., Hammer, S.J. and Smith, N.J. (2001) 'Time trends in autism and in MMR immunisation coverage in california', *Journal of American Medical Association*, 285: 1183-1185.

Danovaro-Holliday, M.C., Wood, A.L. and LeBaron, C.W. (2002) 'Rotavirus vaccine and the news media, 1987-2001', *Journal of American Medical Association*, 287(11): 1455-1458.

Davidson, R., Hunt, K. and Kitzinger, J. (2004) '"Radical blueprint for social change?" Media representations of New Labour's policies on public health' in Seale, C. (ed.) *Health and the Media*. Oxford: Blackwell.

Deacon, D. and Golding, P. (1994) *Taxation and Representation: The Media, Political Communication and the Poll Tax*. London: John Libbey.

Dearing, J.W. (1994) 'Newspaper coverage of maverick science: Creating controversy through balancing', *Public Understanding of Science*, 4: 341-361.

Deer, B. (1998) 'But what if the law got it wrong', *Sunday Times Magazine*, 1 November.

Deer, B. (2004a) 'The truth behind the crisis', *Sunday Times*, 22 February. Page 1.

Deer, B. (2004b) 'Key ally of MMR doctor rejects autism link', *Sunday Times*, 7 March.

Demicheli, V., Jefferson, T., Rivetti, A. and Price, D. (2005) 'Vaccines for measles, mumps and rubella in children', *Cochrane Database Systematic Review*, Oct 19: (4): D004407.

DeWilde, S., Carey, I.M., Richards, N., Hilton, S.R. and Cook, D.G. (2001) 'Do children who become autistic consult more after MMR vaccinations?', *British Journal of General Practice*, March: 226-227.

Donald, A. and Muthu, V. (2002) 'No evidence that MMR vaccine is associated with autism or bowel disease', *Clinical Evidence*, 7: 331-340.

Dornan, C. (1999) 'Some problems in conceptualising the issue of "Science in the media"' in Scanlon, E., et al. (eds.) *Communicating Science: Contexts and Challenges*. London: Routledge.

Dunwoody, S. (1978) *Science Writers at Work*. Research Report No. 7, School of Journalism and Centre for New Communications, Indiana: Indiana University.

Dunwoody, S. (1999) 'Scientists, journalists and the meaning of uncertainty' in Friedman, S.M., Dunwoody, S. and Rogers, C.L. (eds.) *Communicating Uncertainty: Media Coverage of New and Controversial Science.* Hillsdale, New Jersey: Lawrence Erlbaum Associates.

Ehrlich, M.C. (1995) 'The competitive ethos in television newswork', *Critical Studies in Mass Communication,* 12: 196-212.

Ekbom, A., Wakefield, A.J., Zack, M. and Adami, H.O. (1994) 'Perinatal measles infection and subsequent Crohn's disease', *The Lancet,* 344(8921): 508-510.

Eliasoph, N. (1998) *Avoiding Politics.* Cambridge: Cambridge University Press.

Entwistle, V. (1995) 'Reporting research in medical journals and newspapers', *British Medical Journal,* 310(6984): 920-923.

Entwistle, V. and Beaulieu-Hancock, M. (1992) 'Health and medicine coverage in the UK national press', *Public Understanding of Science,* 1: 367-382.

Epstein, S. (1996) *Impure Science.* Berkeley, California: University of California Press.

Ericson, R., Baranek, P. and Chan, J. (1989) *Negotiating Control.* Berkshire: Open University Press.

Evans, G. and Durant, J. (1995) 'The relationship between knowledge and attitudes in the public understanding of science in Britain', *Public Understanding of Science,* 4: 57-74.

Evans, M., Stoddart, H., Condon, L., Freeman, E., Grizzell, M. and Mullen, R. (2001) 'Parents' perspectives on the MMR immunisation: A focus group study', *British Journal of General Practice,* 51: 904-910.

Fairclough, N. (2003) *Media Discourse.* London: Edward Arnold.

Farmelo, G. (1997) 'From big bang to damp squib?' in Levinson, R. and Thomas, J. (eds.) *Science Today: Problem or Crisis?* London: Routledge.

Fitzpatrick, M. (2002) 'Andrew Wakefield: Misguided maverick', www.spiked-online.com/Printable/00000006D8J3.htm (Accessed July 2007).

Fitzpatrick, M. (2004) *MMR and Autism: What Parents Need to Know.* London: Routledge.

Franklin, B. (1999) 'Soft-soaping the public?' in Franklin, B. (ed.) *Social Policy, The Media and Misrepresentation.* London: Routledge.

Frewer, L. and Shepherd, R. (1994) 'Attributing information to different sources: Effects on the perceived qualities of information, on the perceived relevance of information, and on attitude formation', *Public Understanding of Science,* 3: 385-401.

Fursich, E. and Lester, E. (1996) 'Science journalism under scrutiny: A textual analysis of "Science Times", *Critical Studies in Mass Communication,* 13: 24-43.

Galtung, J. and Ruge, M. (1981, original 1965) 'The Structure of Foreign News' in Cohen, S. and Young, J. (eds.) *The Manufacture of News: Deviance, Social Problems and the Mass Media.* London: Constable.

Gangarosa, E. (1998) 'Impact of anti-vaccine movements on pertussis control: The untold story', *The Lancet,* 351: 356-361.

Gans, H.J. (1979) *Deciding What's News.* London: Constable.

Gitlin, T. (1985) *Inside Prime Time.* Berkeley, California: University of California Press.

Glasgow University Media Group. (1976) *Bad News. Vol.1.* London: Routledge and Kegan Paul.

Glasgow University Media Group. (1980) *Bad News. Vol.2, More Bad News.* London: Routledge and Kegan Paul.

Glasgow University Media Group. (1982) *Bad News. Vol.3, Really Bad News.* London: Routledge and Kegan Paul.

Glasser, T.L. (1992) 'Objectivity and news bias' in Cohen, E.D. (ed.) *Philosophical Issues in Journalism.* Oxford: Oxford University Press.

Goldenberg, E. (1975) *Making the Papers.* Lexington, MA: D.C. Heath.

Gosh, P. (2003) *Covering Controversy: Behind the Headline.* Speech given at Science Communication Conference. 22-23 May. Dublin.

Hall, S. (1980) 'Encoding/decoding' in Hall, S., Hobson, D., Lowe, A. and Willis, P. (eds.) *Culture, Media, Language.* London: Hutchinson and Company.

Hall, S., Critcher, C., Jefferson, T., Clarke, J. and Roberts, B. (1978) *Policing the Crisis.* London: Macmillan.

Hallin, D. (1992) 'Sound bite news: Television coverage of elections, 1968-1988', *Journal of Communication,* 42(2): 5-24.

Ham, C. and Alberti, K.G.M.M. (2002) 'The medical profession, the public and the government', *British Medical Journal,* 324: 838 -842.

Hansen, A. (1994) 'Journalistic practices and science reporting in the British press', *Public Understanding of Science,* 3: 111-134.

Hansen, A. and Dickinson, R. (1992) 'Science coverage in the British mass media: Media output and source input', *Communications: European Journal of Communication Research,* 17(3): 365-377.

Harcup, T. and O'Neill, D. (2001) 'What is news? Galtung and Ruge revisited', *Journalism Studies,* 2(2): 261-280.

Hargreaves, I. and Ferguson, G. (2000) *Who's Misunderstanding Whom?* London: ESRC.

Hargreaves, I., Lewis, J. and Speers, T. (2003) *Towards a Better Map: Science, the Public and the Media.* London: ESRC.

Hargreaves, I. and Thomas, J. (2002) *New News, Old News.* London: ITC/BSC.

Harrabin, R., Coote, A. and Allen, J. (2003) *Health in the News.* London: King's Fund.

Henderson, L. and Kitzinger, J. (1999) 'The human drama of genetics: "Hard" and "soft" media representations of inherited breast cancer', *Sociology of Health and Illness,* 21(5): 560-578.

Henwood, F., Wyatt, S., Hart, A. and Smith, J. (2004) '"Ignorance is bliss sometimes": Constraints on the emergence of the "Informed Patient" in the changing landscapes of health information' in Seale, C. (ed.) *Health and the Media.* Oxford: Blackwell.

Herman, E. and Chomsky, N. (1988) *Manufacturing Consent.* New York: Pantheon.

Hijmans, E., Pleijter, A. and Wester, F. (2003) 'Covering scientific research in Dutch newspapers', *Science Communication,* 25(2): 153-176.

Hobson-West, P. (2003) 'Understanding vaccine resistance: Moving beyond risk', *Health, Risk and Society,* 5(3): 273-283.

Honda H., Shimizu Y. and Rutter, M. (2005) 'No effect of MMR withdrawal on the incidence of autism: A total population study', *Journal of Child Psychology and Psychiatry*, 46(6): 572-579.

Horlick-Jones, T. (2004) 'Experts in risk?...Do they exist?', *Health, Risk and Society*, 6(2): 107-114.

Hornig-Priest, S. (1999) 'Securing public debate on biotechnology' in Scanlon, E. et al. (eds.) *Communicating Science: Contexts and Challenges*. London: Routledge.

Horton, R. (2003) *Second Opinion: Doctors, Diseases and Decisions in Modern Medicine*. London: Granta.

Horton, R. (2004a) *MMR Science and Fiction*. London: Granta.

Horton, R. (2004b) 'The lessons of MMR', *The Lancet*, 363 (9411): 747.

INRA Europe (2000) *Eurobarometer 52.1:The Europeans and Biotechnology*. www.europa.eu.int/comm/research/pdf/eurobarometer-en.pdf (Accessed November 2006).

Jewell, D. (2001) 'Editorial', *British Journal of General Practice*, 51: 875-876.

Jones, N. (2003) 'Television impartiality or biased news?', *Campaign for Press and Broadcasting Freedom*, http://keywords.dsvr.co.uk/freepress/body.phtml?category=&id=563 (Accessed November 2006).

Journalism Training Forum (2002) *Journalists at Work*. UK: Publishing Industry National Training Organisation and Skillset.

Karpf, A. (1988) *Doctoring the Media*. London: Routledge.

Katz, E., and Lazarsfeld, P. (1955) *Personal Influence*. New York: The Free Press.

Kaye, J.A., Melero-Montes, M. and Jick, H. (2001) 'Mumps, measles and rubella vaccine and the incidence of autism recorded by general practitioners: A time trend analysis', *British Medical Journal*, 322: 460-463.

Kitzinger, J. (1998) 'The gender politics of news production' in Carter, C., Branston, G. and Allan, S. (eds.) *News, Gender and Power*. London: Routledge.

Kitzinger, J. (1999a) 'Researching risk and the media', *Health, Risk and Society*, 1(1): 55-69.

Kitzinger, J. (1999b) 'A sociology of media power, key issues in audience reception research' in Philo, G. (ed.) *Message Received*. UK: Longman.

Kitzinger, J. (2004) *Framing Abuse: Media Influence and Public Understandings of Sexual Violence Against Children*. London: Pluto.

Kitzinger, J. and Reilly, L. (1997) 'The rise and fall of risk reporting', *European Journal of Communication*, 12 (3): 319-350.

Klaidman, S. (1990) 'How well the media report health risk', *Daedalus*, 4: 119-132.

Kulenkampff, M., Schwartzman, J.S. and Wilson, J. (1974) 'Neurological complications of pertussis inoculation', *Archives of Disease in Childhood*, 49: 46-49.

Kumar, D. (2007) *Outside the Box: Corporate Media, Globalization, and the UPS Strike*. Champaign, Illinois: University of Illinois Press.

Labinger, J. (2001) 'Let's not get too agreeable' in Labinger, J. and Collins, H. (eds.) *The One Culture?* Chicago: University of Chicago Press.

Langer, J. (1998) *Tabloid Television: Popular Journalism and The 'Other News'*. London: Routledge.

Lantz, J.C. and Lanier, W.L. (2002) 'Observations from the Mayo Clinic national conference on medicine and the media', *Mayo Clinic Proc.*, 77: 1306-1311.

Law, J. (2006) *Big Pharma: How the World's Drug Companies Control Illness*. London: Constable.

Le Fanu, J. (1999) 'The fall of medicine', *Prospect*, July: 28-31.

Levi, R. (2001) *Medical Journalism: Exposing Fact, Fiction, Fraud*. Ames, Iowa: Iowa State University Press.

Lewis, J. (1991) *The Ideological Octopus: An Exploration of Television and its Audience*. London: Routledge.

Lewis, J. (2001) *Constructing Public Opinion: How Political Elites Do What They Like and Why We Seem To Go Along With It*. New York: Columbia University Press.

Lewis, J. and Wahl-Jorgensen, K. (2005) 'Active citizen or couch potato? Journalism and public opinion' in Allan, S. (ed.) *Journalism: Critical Issues*. Berkshire: Open University Press.

Lewis, J. Wahl-Jorgensen, K. and Inthorn, S. (2005) *Citizens or Consumers? What the Media Tells Us About Public Participation*. Berkshire: Open University Press.

Lichtenberg, J. (1996) 'In defence of objectivity revisited' in Curran, J. and Gurevitch, M. (eds.) *Mass Media and Society: Second Edition*. London: Arnold.

Limoges, C. (1993) 'Expert knowledge and decision-making in controversy contexts', *Public Understanding of Science*, 2: 417-426.

Livingstone, S. and Lunt, P. (1994) *Talk on Television: Audience Participation and Public Debates*. London: Routledge.

Logan, R. A. (1991) 'Popularisation versus secularization: Media coverage of health' in Wilkins, L. and Patterson, P. (eds.) *Risky Business: Communicating Issues of Science, Risk and Public Policy*. Westport, CT: Greenwood Press.

Lupton, D. (1998) 'Medicine and health care in popular media' in Petersen, A. and Waddell, C. (eds.) *Health Matters*. Berkshire: Open University Press.

Lupton, D. (2003) 'Representations of medicine, illness and disease in elite and popular culture' in Lupton, D. (ed.) *Medicine as Culture*. London: Sage.

Lupton, D. and Mclean, J. (1998) 'Representing doctors: Discourses and images in the Australian press', *Social Studies of Medicine*, 46(8): 947-958.

MacDowell, I. (compiled by) (1992) *Reuters Handbook for Journalists*. London: Butterworth Heinemann.

Madsen, K.M., Hviid, A., Vestergaard, M., Schendel, D., Wohlfahrt, J., Thorsen, P., Olsen, J. and Melbye, M. (2002) 'A population-based study of measles, mumps and rubella vaccination and autism', *New England Journal of Medicine*, 347: 1477-1482.

Maier, S.R. (2002). 'Getting it right? Not in 59 percent of stories', *Newspaper Research Journal*, 23: 10–24.

Malcolm, J. (1983) *The Journalist and the Murderer*. London: Granta.

Manning, P. (2001) *News and News Sources: A Critical Introduction*. London: Sage.

Mason, B.W. and Donnelly, P.D. (2000) 'Impact of a local newspaper campaign on the uptake of measles, mumps and rubella vaccine', *Journal of Epidemiological Community Health*, 54: 473-474.

Matheson, D. (2005) *Media Discourses: Analysing Media Texts*. Berkshire Open University Press.

Mayhew, L.H. (1997) *The New Public: Professional Communication and the Means of Social Influence*. Cambridge: Cambridge University Press.

Mazur, A. (1981) 'Media coverage and public opinion on scientific controversies', *Journal of Communication*, 31: 106-115.

Mencher, M. (1997) *News Reporting and Writing*. Madison, WI: Brown and Benchmark Publishers.

Merritt, D. (1995) *Public Journalism and Public Life: Why Telling the News is Not Enough*. Hillsdale, New Jersey: Lawrence Erlbaum Associates.

Miller, D. (1999) 'Mediating science' in Scanlon, E. et al. (eds.) *Communicating Science: Contexts and Challenges*. London: Routledge.

Miller, D., Kitzinger, J., Williams, K. and Beharrell, P. (1998) *The Circuit of Mass Communication*. London: Sage.

Miller, D. and Reilly, J. (1995) 'Making an issue of food safety: The media, pressure groups and the public sphere' in Maurer, D. and Sobal, J. (eds.) *Eating Agendas: Food and Nutrition as Social Problems*. New York: Aldine de Gruyter.

Miller, M.M. and Riechert, B.P. (2000) 'Interest group strategies and journalistic norms' in Allan, S., Adam, B. and Carter, C. (eds.) *Environmental Risks and the Media*. London: Routledge.

Molitor, F. (1993) 'Accuracy in science news reporting by newspapers: The case of aspirin for the prevention of heart attacks', *Health Communication*, 5(3): 209-224.

Mormont, M. and Dasnoy, C. (1995) 'Source strategies and the mediatization of climate change', *Media, Culture and Society*, 17: 49-64.

Morris, A. and Aldulaimi, D. (2002) 'New evidence for a viral pathogenic mechanism for new variant inflammatory bowel disease and development disorder', *Molecular Pathology*, 55(2): 83.

MRC (2001) *MRC Review of Autism Research: Epidemiology and Causes*. London: Medical Research Council.

Murch, S., Thomson, M. and Walker-Smith, J. (1998) 'Autism, inflammatory bowel disease and MMR vaccine', *The Lancet*, 351: 9106.

Murch, S. (2003) 'Separating inflammation from speculation in autism', *The Lancet*, 362: 1498-1499.

Murch, S., Anthony, A., Casson, D., Malik, M., Berelowitz, M., Dhillon, A., Thomson, M., Valentine, A., Davies, S. and Walker-Smith, J. (2004) 'Retraction of interpretation', *The Lancet*, 363: 750.

Mythen, G. (2004) *Ulrich Beck: A Critical Introduction to the Risk Society*. London: Pluto Press.

Nelkin, D. (1987) *Selling Science. How the Press Covers Science and Technology*. (first edition) New York, New York: W.H. Freeman and Company.

Newman, T.B. (2003) 'The power of stories over statistics', *British Medical Journal*, 327: 1424-1427.

Offit, P.A. and Coffin, S.E. (2003) 'Communicating science to the public: MMR vaccine and autism', *Vaccine*, 22: 1-6.

Palmer, J. (2000) *Spinning Into Control: News Values and Source Strategies*. London: Leicester University Press.

Passwell, J. (1999) 'MMR vaccination, Crohn's disease and autism: A real or imagined "Stomach Ache/Headache"', *Israeli Medical Association Journal*, 1: 176-177.

Patja, A., Davidkin, I., Kurki, T., Kallio, M.J.T. and Valle, M.H.P. (2002) 'Serious adverse events after MMR vaccination during a 14-year prospective follow-up', *Paediatric Infectious Disease Journal*, 19: 1127-1134.

Peltola, H., Heinonen, D.P., Valle, M., Paunio, M., Virtanen, M., Karanko, V. and Cantell K. (1994) 'The elimination of indigenous measles, mumps and rubella from Finland by a 12 year old dose vaccination program', *New England Journal of Medicine*, 331: 1397-1402.

Peltola, H., Patja, A., Leinikki, P., Valle, M., Davidkin, I. and Paunio, M. (1998) 'No evidence for measles, mumps and rubella vaccine-associated inflammatory bowel disease or autism in a 14-year prospective study', *The Lancet*, 351: 1327-1328.

Petts, J. and Niemeyer, S. (2004) 'Health risk communication and amplification: Learning from the MMR vaccination controversy', *Health, Risk and Society*, 6(1): 7-23.

Phillips, D.P., Kanter, E.J., Bednarczyck, B. and Tastad, P.L. (1991) 'Importance of the lay press in the transmission of medical knowledge to the scientific community', *New England Journal of Medicine*, 325: 1180-1183.

Philo, G. (ed.) (1999) *Message Received*. Harlow: Longman.

Pollock, A. (2004) *NHS PLC: The Privatisation of Our Healthcare*. London: Verso.

Ramsay, M.E., Yarwood, J., Lewis, D., Campbell H. and White J.M. (2002) 'Parental confidence in measles, mumps and rubella vaccine: Evidence from vaccine coverage and attitudinal surveys', *British Journal of General Practice*, 52 (484): 912-916.

Reed, R. (2001) '(Un-) professional discourse?', *Journalism*, 2(3): 279-298.

Resenberger, B. (1997) 'Covering science for newspapers' in Blum, D. and Knudson, M. (eds.) *A Field Guide for Science Writers*. Oxford: Oxford University Press.

Rimal, R., Flora, J.A., and Schooler, C. (1999) 'Achieving improvements in overall health orientation', *Communication Research*, 26(3): 322-348.

Rogers, C.L. (1999) 'The importance of understanding audiences' in Friedman, S.M., Dunwoody, S. and Rogers, C.L. (eds.) *Communicating Uncertainty: Media Coverage of New and Controversial Science*. Hillsdale, New Jersey: Lawrence Erlbaum Associates.

Rogers, A. and Pilgrim, D. (1995) 'The risk of resistance: Perspectives on the mass childhood immunisation programme', in Gabe, J. (ed.) *Medicine, Health and Risk*. Oxford: Blackwell.

Rowe, R., Tilbury, F., Rapley, M. and O'Ferrall, I. (2004) "'About a year before the breakdown I was having symptoms": Sadness, pathology and the Australian newspaper media' in Seale, C. (ed.) *Health and the Media*. Oxford: Blackwell.

Royal Society (2006) *Science and the Public Interest*. London: Royal Society.

Schudson, M. (1978) *Discovering the News: A Social History of American Newspapers*. New York: Basic Books.

Seale, C. (2002) *Media and Health*. London: Sage.

Seale, C. (2004) 'Health and the media' in Seale, C. (ed.) *Health and the Media*. Oxford: Blackwell.

Seymour-Ure, C. (1977) 'Science and medicine and the press' in Boyd-Barrett, O., Seymour-Ure, C. and Tunstall, J. (eds.) *Studies on the Press*. Cardiff: HMO.

Sheridan Burns, L. (2002) *Understanding Journalism*. London: Sage.

Singer, E. (1990) 'A question of accuracy: How journalists and scientists report research on hazards', *Journal of Communication*, 40(4): 102-116.

Singer, E. and Endreny, P. (1987) 'Reporting hazards: Their benefits and costs', *Journal of Communication*, 37(3): 10-26.

Singer, E. and Endreny, P. (1993) *Reporting on Risk: How the Mass Media Portray Accidents, Diseases, Disasters and Other Hazards*. New York: Sage.

Sokal, A. (1996) 'Transgressing the boundaries: Towards a transformative hermeneutics of quantum gravity', *Social Text*, 46/47: 217-252.

Soley, L. (1992) *The News Shapers*. New York: Praeger.

Soley, L. (1994) 'Pundits in print', *Newspaper Research Journal*, 15: 65-75.

Starkey, G. (2006) *Balance and Bias in Journalism*. New York: Palgrave.

Steele, J. (1995) 'Experts and the operational bias of television news: The case of the Persian Gulf War', *Journalism and Mass Communication Quarterly*, 72(4): 799-812.

Stocking, S.H. (1999) 'How journalists deal with uncertainty' in Friedman, S.M., Dunwoody, S. and Rogers, C.L. (eds.) *Communicating Uncertainty: Media Coverage of New and Controversial Science*. Hillsdale, New Jersey: Lawrence Erlbaum Associates.

Taylor, B., Miller, E., Farrington, C.P., Petropoulos, M.C., Favot-Mayaud, I., Li, J. and Waight, P.A. (1999) 'Autism and measles, mumps and rubella vaccine: No epidemiological evidence for a causal association', *The Lancet*, 353(9169): 2026-2029.

Taylor, B. Miller, E., Lingam, R., Andrews, N., Simmons, A. and Stowe, J. (2002) 'Measles, mumps and rubella vaccination and bowel problems or developmental regression in children with autism: Population study', *British Medical Journal*, 324: 393-396.

Thomas, J. (1997) 'Informed ambivalence' in Levinson, R. and Thomas, J. (eds.) *Science Today: Problem or Crisis?* London: Routledge.

Thompson, N.P., Montgomery, S.M., Pounder, R.E. and Wakefield, A.J. (1995) 'Is measles vaccination a risk factor for inflammatory bowel disease?', *The Lancet*, 345(8957):1071-1074.

Tuchman, G. (1972) 'Objectivity as strategic ritual: An examination of newsmen's notions of objectivity', *American Journal of Sociology*, 77: 660-679 in Tumber, H. (ed.) *News: A Reader*. Oxford: Oxford University Press.

Tunstall, J. (1971) *Journalists at Work*. London: Sage.

Uhlmann, V., Martin, C., Sheils, O., Pilkington, L., Silva, I., Killalea, A., Murch, S., Walker-Smith, J., Thomson M., Wakefield, A.J. and O'Leary, J.J. (2002) 'Potential viral pathogenic mechanism for new variant inflammatory bowel disease', *Molecular Pathology*, 55: 84-90.

Van Dijk, T. (1991) *Racism in the Press: Critical Studies in Racism and Migration*. London: Routledge.

Wakefield, A.J. (2003) Interview on BBC Radio Programme *Today*. October 31.

Wakefield, A.J., Anthony, A., Murch, S., Thomson, M., Montgomery, S.M., Davies, S., O'Leary, J.J., Berelowitz, M. and Walker-Smith, J.A. (2000) 'Enterocolitis in children with developmental disorders', *American Journal of Gastroenterology*, 95: 2285-2295.

Wakefield, A.J., and Montgomery S.M. (1999) 'Autism, viral infection and measles mumps, rubella vaccination', *Israeli Medical Association Journal*, 1: 183-187.

Wakefield, A.J., Murch S., Anthony, A., Linnell, J., Casson, D.M., Malik, M., Berelowitz, M., Dhillon, A.P., Thomson, M.A., Harvey, P., Valentine, A., Davies, S.E. and Walker-Smith, J. (1998) 'Ileal-lymphoid-nodular hyperplasia, non-specific colitis, and pervasive developmental disorder in children', *The Lancet*, 351(9103): 637-641.

Weimann, G., Tustin, D., Vuuren, D. and Joubert, J. (2007) 'Looking for opinion leaders: Traditional vs. modern measures in traditional societies', *International Journal of Public Opinion*, 119(2):173-190.

Williams, C., Kitzinger, J. and Henderson, L. (2003) 'Envisaging the embryo in stem cell research: Rhetorical strategies and media reporting of the ethical debates', *Sociology of Health and Illness*, 25(7):793-814.

Wynne, B. (1989) 'Sheep farming after Chernobyl: A case study in communicating scientific information', *Environmental Magazine*, 31(2): 33-39.

Zelizer, B. (1997) 'Journalists as interpretive communities' in Berkowitz, D. (ed.) *Social Meanings of News: A Text-Reader*. London: Sage.

Index

C

D

M

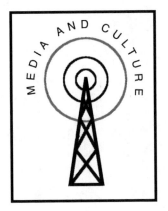

Sut Jhally & Justin Lewis
General Editors

This series publishes works on media and culture, focusing on research embracing a variety of critical perspectives. The series is particularly interested in promoting theoretically informed empirical work using both quantitative and qualitative approaches. Although the focus is on scholarly research, the series aims to speak beyond a narrow, specialist audience.

ALSO AVAILABLE

- Michael Morgan, Editor
  Against the Mainstream: The Selected Works of George Gerbner

- Edward Herman
  The Myth of the Liberal Media: An Edward Herman Reader

- Robert Jensen
  Writing Dissent: Taking Radical Ideas from the Margins to the Mainstream

To order other books in this series, please contact our Customer Service Department at:

(800) 770-LANG (within the U.S.)
(212) 647-7706 (outside the U.S.)
(212) 647-7707 FAX

or browse online by series at:
WWW.PETERLANG.COM